TAICHI WALKING FOR SENIORS

Unlock Japanese Interval Walking & Tai Chi to Burn Fat, Calm the Mind, andReclaim Energy in Just 30 Minutes a Day — No Running, No Gym, No Stress.

Dear Reader.

Thank you for purchasing this book and for taking the first step toward a more grounded, energetic, and resilient version of yourself.

TAICHI Walking For Seniors was written with you in mind: Whether you' re over 40, starting over, feeling disconnected from your body, or simply craving a routine that regenerates rather than drains you, you' re in the right place.

Every page is designed to convey support, flexibility, and strength.Here are some tips to get you started:

> Move gently. You don't have to be fit or coordinated. This book respects your rhythm, your pace, your body.
> Stay safe. Always listen to your body. If you feel discomfort,take a break. And consult your doctor before starting nea movements.
> Adapt to your needs. You' ll find modifications for different ages and body types, and simple adjustments for every energy level.
> Track your progress. Use the included tracker to celebrate your progress. True healing happens in small, daily steps.

Above all: be kind to yourself.

This book isn't about perfection, but about connection. With your breath. With your steps. With the strength that's still within you.

Let's walk this healing journey together.

You' re not starting over. You' re moving forward.

With gratitude and encouragement.

TAICHI WALKING FOR SENIORS: COMPLETE INDEX

CHAPTER 1-Why Walking Alone Isn't Always Enough ·················· Pag.7
· The Hidden Problem with "Just Walk More"
· What's Missing? Rhythm. breath. Awareness.
· Stop "Just Walking." Start healing.

Your Body Is Not Broken, It's Out Of Rhythm ························· Pag.10
· You're Not Broken. You're Desynchronized.
· The Problem Is Not Age-It's Disconnection
· Rhythm= Regulation
· Reclaiming Your Inner Clock

CHAPTER 2. The Origins: East Meets East ····················· Pag.12
·CN Tai Chi Walking-Movement as Meditation
· JP Japanese Interval Walking-Power Meets Precision
· Why "East Meets East" Works
· The healing Walk Method is Born

The 3 Core Pillars Of The healing Walk Method ··············· Pag.14
· Pillar 1: Rhythmic Movement
· Pillar 2: Conscious Breathing
· Pillar 3: Mindful Posture

Why This Method Works Especially For Women Over 40 ············· Pag.17
· What's Really Going On After 40?
· A Method That Aligns with the Female Body

CHAPTER 3-Getting Started: Your healing Walk Plan ············ Pag.19
· What You Need (And Don't Need) To Begin
· Indoor vs. Outdoor: What's Better?
· What If I'm Out of Shape or Injured?

The Optimal Walking Schedule For healing, Balance, And Energy ········ Pag.22
· The healing Walk Weekly Blueprint
· Weekly Goals-What to Expect

Preparing Your Mind: Setting The Intention Before You Step ············ Pag.24
· 3-Step Pre-Walk Intention ritual (Takes 2 Minutes or Less)

Walking Into Flow: How To Feel Your Body Instead Of Fighting It ········ Pag.26
· What Is Flow-and Why Does It Matter?
· How to Walk Into Flow-5 Simple Triggers

CHAPTER 4. The Basic healing Walk Sequence (Step- By- Step) .... Pag. 28
HEALING WALK-FULL SEquence (15-30 MINUTES)
　①Grounding (2-3 minutes)
　②Gentle Start (3 minutes)
　③Rhythm & breath Phase (12-20 minutes)
　④Mind- Body Integration (2-3 minutes)

Breathwork Techniques That Unlock Deeper healing .... Pag. 31
BREATH TECHNIQUES FOR HEALING WALKS:
　　1. The 3:3 Walking Breath
　　2. The 4:4 Deep healing Breath
　　3. The 2:6 Detox breath

　· **When to Use Each breath** .... Pag. 33
Posture Reset: Aligning Your Body for Long- TermMobility&Grace .... Pag. 35
　· **The 5- Point Posture Reset (While Walking)** .... Pag. 35
THE WALKING FLOW PROTOCOL (Your Daily 15-30 Minute Template)
.... Pag.38
　· Option A-15- Minute Reset (Short & Powerful)
　· Option B-30- Minute Transformation Walk
　· Weekly healing Walk Flow

CHAPTER 5. Japanese Interval Walking & Core Tai Chi Form Pag.40
· Japanese Interval Walking (JIW): What It Is And Why It Works
　· Clinical Results That matter
　· Why It Works Especially Well for Women 40+

How To Practice Japanese Interval Walking .... Pag. 41
　· The Simple Rule
　· How Fast Is"Brisk"?
　· Your First 14- Day Japanese Walking Plan

THE CORE TAI CHI WALKING FORM Step- By- Step Breakdown .... Pag. 45
　· STRUCTURE OVERVIEW:5 ELEMENTS
　· STEP-BY-STEP WALKING FORM:

COMMON MISTAKES TO AVOID During Tai Chi Walking Practice Pag.47
Modifications For Different Ages & Body Types Pag.49

CHAPTER 6. Suggested Routine. .... Pag. 51
· Tai Chi Walking+ Japanese Interval Walking (JIW) Combinations
　· 1).15/15 FUSION Routine
　· 2).10/10/10 TRIPLE ROUTINE
　· 3). ALTERNATING DAYS METHOD

· **Emotional Awareness Through Each Step** .... Pag. 52
　· 3 Types of Emotional Walking Practices
　　　1. Calm Walk (For Anxiety, Overthinking)
　　　2. Fire Walk (For Sadness, Stuck Energy)
　　　3. Flow Walk (For Reconnection, Presence)

- **Breath-Based Emotional Detox** ··· Pag.54
  ○ Breath Ratios: The Secret Sauce
  ○ Your 7-Day Breathwalk Reset Plan

CHAPTER 7. The Integrative Reset ··································· Pag.58
· How This Reset Works
·DAY1-Grounding Your Energy
·DAY 2-Igniting Your Metabolism
·DAY3-Clearing Mental Fog
·DAY 4-Releasing Emotional Tension
·DAY5-Building Inner Strength
·DAY6-Healing Walk
·DAY 7-Integration+ Gratitude

CHAPTER 8. Walking Beyond Weight Loss···························· Pag.61
· The Spiritual and Hormonal Intelligence of Walking
  ○ Walking Regulates Your Hormones — Silently, Powerfully
· Walking as a Moving Meditation
· Spiritual Walking Practices
   1. The"Presence Path"
   2. The Moonlight Release
   3. The Gratitude Spiral

CHAPTER 9-WALKING AS A LIFELONG HABIT···················· Pag.65
· Building Your Unshakeable Walking Identity
· The Habit Loop of Walking
· The 5-Minute Minimum Method
· Walking Identity Affirmations
· Weekly Walking Templates

CHAPTER 10 – BONUS PROTOCOLS: The Hidden Power Of Walking

AsEnergy Medicine···Pag.67
·**QIGONG WALKING-The Ancient Flow in Motion**
  ○ Basic Qigong Walking Technique-5 Steps
  ○ Qigong Walking Vs Tai Chi Walking (Includes Comparison Table)
  ○ HOW TO BLEND TAI CHI, QIGONG, AND JIW

- **Silent Walking-The Mirror Of The Mind** ····························· Pag69
·EMOTIONAL LOOP RESET-The Interrupt + Replace Model
· Summary Chart: Bonus Protocols

30-DAY HEALING WALK PLAN (CALENDAR)···················· Pag.70
  ○ WEEK1: AWARENESS (Days 1-7)
  ○ WEEK 2:RHYTHM (Days 8-14)
  ○ WEEK 3:ENERGY (Days 15-21)
  ○ WEEK 4: INTEGRATION (Days 22-30)

CHAPTER 11. How To Teach Others & Form Walking Groups .... **Pag. 72**
· Why Teach or Walk in Groups?
· Benefits of Group Walking Practice
· How to Start Teaching or Leading
· Create a Simple Structure
· Tips for Success

BUNUS & APPENDICES:
  BUNUS- WALKING JOURNAL TEMPLATE + HOW TO LEAVE A POWERFUL REVIEW .... **Pag. 74**
   · Why a Walking Journal Changes Everything
   · Daily Walk Journal Template:
BUNUS-MUSIC & INTERVAL SYNCING **Pag.76**
  · WHY BPM MATTERS (BPM = Beats Per Minute)
  ·INTERVAL MUSIC SYNCING
  ·SUGGESTED SPOTIFY PLAYLISTS
· **HOW TO TEACH OTHERS & FORM WALKING GROUPS (AdvancedTips)** **Pag.77**
  · START SMALL: THE"MICRO-CLASS"METHOD
  ·FORMING A WALKING GROUP
·**REFERENCES: Studies, Sources, and Traditions** **Pag.78**
  · Tai Chi Walking
  · Japanese Interval Walking (JIW)
  · Qigong Walking
  · Mind- Body & Behavior Science
· **Cultural Acknowledgments** .... **Pag. 80**

CHAPTER 1

Why Walking Alone Isn't Always Enough.

Walking is often praised as the perfect exercise: low-impact, accessible, and free. For decades, we've been told, "Just walk more and you'll feel better." But if you're here, chances are you've already tried that. You've walked the same path around your neighborhood. You've tracked your steps, watched the numbers go up... and still felt like something was missing.
That's because walking, by itself, doesn't automatically lead to healing.
Let's be honest: many of you are walking while still carrying anxiety, fatigue, hormonal imbalances, or joint pain. The steps may be happening, but the transformation isn't. It's like having the right vehicle... but no map, no fuel, and no destination.
This is why the way you walk matters just as much as walking itself.
The Hidden Problem with "Just Walk More".
Modern fitness advice often treats all movement as equal. But walking while scrolling on your phone, or power walking while mentally running through your to-do list, isn't going to bring you the emotional reset, metabolic boost, or physical healing you truly need.
In fact, walking without presence or rhythm can become just another task—— another thing you check off, but never truly feel.
That's why many people give up.
That's why weight doesn't drop.
That's why stress lingers, even after the walk.

What's Missing? Rhythm. Breath. Awareness.
When we look at ancient movement practices from Japan and China, like Japanese Interval Walking and Tai Chi Walking, a very different picture emerges:
    Movement isn't random—— it's structured
    Breath isn't forgotten—— it leads the motion
    Mindfulness isn't optional—— it's the core engine
This is why these practices deliver more than just fitness—— they activate your nervous system, metabolism, emotions, and balance, all at once.

A Quick Analogy:
Imagine two people walking side by side.
One is listening to stressful news and rushing.
The other is synced with her breath, walking with mindful posture, moving in intervals of energy and rest.
Same number of steps. completely different effect on the body.

Stop "Just Walking." Start healing.
If you've been walking for months —— or even years —— without:
- Losing the stubborn belly fat
- Feeling lighter in your joints
- Sleeping better
- Reducing anxiety or brain fog
- Regaining your energy...

… it's not your fault.
You don't need to push harder. You need to walk differently.
And that's exactly what you're going to learn in this book.

This book isn't about walking more.
It's about walking with purpose, rhythm, breath, and healing awareness.
That's how you burn fat, calm your nervous system, and rewire your energy at the same time.

ate known as sympathetic dominance (fight or flight).Now here's the good news:
Intentional walking with rhythmic breathing activates the parasympathetic nervous system, also known as the" rest and repair" mode. This shift is measurable:
- Heart rate slows,
- Breath deepens,
- Muscle tension reduces,
- Inflammation markers drop,
- Cortisol (stress hormone) decreases.

This is the state where healing happens—— and it can be accessed by simply walking… the right way.
The breath- Walk Connection.
Breathing is the only autonomic function you can control at will. That makes it a powerful bridge between your conscious mind and your body. When you synchronize your breath with your steps—— like in Tai Chi Walking or JapaneseInterval Walking—— you create a rhythmic loop that calms the mind while energizing the body.This creates:
- Greater oxygen efficiency,

Improved cardiovascular performance,
Reduced fatigue and anxiety.

Example:
Breathing in for 3 steps and out for 3 steps is a basic pattern in Japanese Interval Walking. When done consistently, it resets your internal rhythm, especially in women over 40 experiencing hormonal imbalance or adrenal fatigue.

SCIENCE SNAPSHOT: Interval Walking & Longevity.
A study published by the Japanese team at Shinshu University showed that alternating 3 minutes of brisk walking with 3 minutes of slow walking, five times a week, led to:
Increased VO_2 max (aerobic capacity).
Improved insulin sensitivity.
Reduced visceral fat.
Enhanced mood and memory in older adults.

These results weren't from running or intense cardio. Just interval- based walking with a conscious breath pattern.
Walking becomes healing when it's intentional. breath is the medicine. Rhythm is the carrier.

Tai Chi Principles: Movement as Energy Flow.
Tai Chi isn't just slow motion exercise—— it's a system of internal alignment.
When applied to walking:
Your posture elongates the spine,
Your steps glide rather than stomp,
Your arms swing with gentle circular motion,
Your breath leads, your body follows.

This brings a unique benefit: joint relief without stagnation. That's why Tai Chi Walking is often used in rehab settings—— it stimulates flow without impact.

Combining Both = Dual Activation

Practice	Benefit
Japanese Interval Walking	Activates metabolism, burns fat, builds cardiovascular strength
Tai Chi Walking	Calms the nervous system, reduces joint stress, improves balance

Combining them creates a method that heals while it energizes, and tones while it soothes——ideal for people over 40 who want results without punishment.
You're not just walking anymore.
You're training your brain, healing your hormones, and reprogramming your energy—— all at once.

Your Body Is Not Broken, It's Out Of Rhythm.

If you've ever felt like your body is betraying you—— you're not alone.
The fatigue.
The bloating.
The foggy mornings.
The aches that weren't there last year...
Many of you, especially over 40, may have started to believe:
"Maybe I'm just getting old."
"Maybe this is the new normal."
"Maybe I'm broken."
Stop. That belief is the first thing we're going to dismantle.
You're Not Broken. You're Desynchronized.
What if your body wasn't failing... but simply out of sync?
Think of your body like a complex orchestra. When each section—— your heart, hormones, lungs, joints, and brain—— plays in rhythm, the result is harmony: energy, clarity, vitality.
But what happens when:

- Your sleep is off
- Your breathing is shallow
- Your stress is constant
- Your movement is mechanical
- Your pace is dictated by everything except your own rhythm?

You get noise. You get chaos instead of harmony. And your body reacts with pain, inflammation, and burnout.

The Problem Is Not Age— It's Disconnection.

Many women and men over 40 are told, "Just accept the changes." But what if these changes are signals—— not of decline, but of misalignment?
Let's look at a few real-life scenarios from our buyer persona profiles:

- Maria, 52: She walks daily but wakes up feeling drained. Her hormones are off, but her doctor says she's "fine."
- Denise, 47: She tries high-intensity workouts but ends up more anxious and inflamed. She's "doing everything right," but nothing changes.
- Elena, 61: She's recovering from an injury, afraid to move. She misses feeling vibrant but doesn't trust her body anymore.

In all these cases, the body is asking for reconnection, not punishment. And that's what this method gives you: a new language to speak with your body.

Rhythm = Regulation

Modern life fragments us. But ancient wisdom—— and now modern science —— shows us that restoring rhythm is the fastest way to:
- Balance cortisol and adrenaline,
- Reset sleep-wake cycles,
- Reduce inflammation markers,
- Improve digestion and immunity,
- Boost mitochondrial energy.

Walking in rhythm, with breath, awareness, and structure, re-entrains the body's systems to move together again. The heart and lungs start to collaborate. The nervous system downshifts. Your digestion improves, your focus returns, and the fatigue starts to lift.

This isn't magic. It's biology——when you bring back the beat.
Reclaiming Your Inner Clock.
The healing Walk Method isn't just a fitness tool.
It's a reset button for your internal rhythms——hormonal, metabolic, emotional, and physical.

We'll show you:
- How to walk in sync with your natural energy cycles,
- How to train your circadian and ultradian rhythms,
- How to rewire your internal GPS to trust your body again.

Because once your body remembers its own rhythm...it knows exactly how to heal itself.

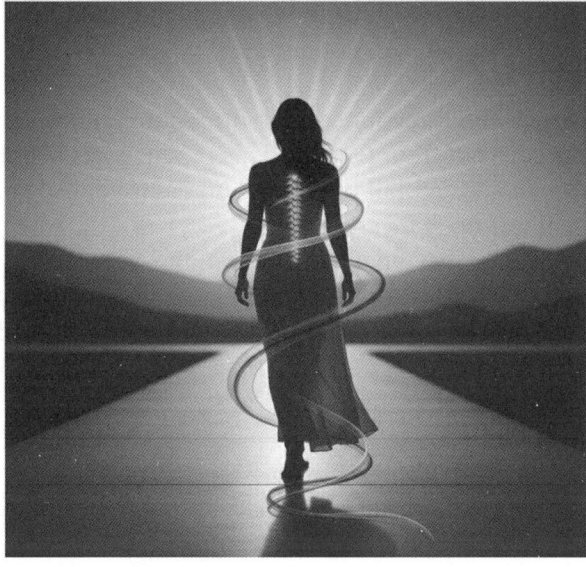

CHAPTER 2

The Origins: East Meets East.

What happens when two ancient cultures, each with their own rich traditions of movement,healing, and mindfulness, unknowingly align on the same core truth?
You get The healing Walk Method.

This chapter explores how the practices of Tai Chi Walking (China) and Japanese IntervalWalking (Japan)—— though developed in different eras, for different reasons—— share an underlying rhythm, a respect for the body, and a path to healing that modern science is just now beginning to validate.

CN Tai Chi Walking-Movement as Meditation.
Tai Chi Chuan originated in ancient China as a martial art, but quickly evolved into a form of" moving meditation" practiced for longevity, balance, and internal harmony.

While many associate Tai Chi with slow arm movements and graceful sequences, there's a lesser-known but deeply powerful element: Tai Chi Walking.
- Rooted in Daoist philosophy,
- Focused on internal balance, posture, and breath,
- Movements are circular, intentional, and grounded,
- Steps are slow, deliberate, and in sync with breath.
- Energy (qi) is cultivated, not drained

Tai Chi Walking is about reconnecting with your center. It trains you to walk from your core,not from tension. This practice has been shown to:
- Improve balance and fall prevention in older adults
- Enhance mind-body awareness
- Activate deep parasympathetic relaxation

But here's the key: it's slow. Beautiful, but slow. Many modern walkers—— especially those seeking fat loss, energy, and dynamic health—— feel they need more activation.
And that's where Japan steps in.

JP Japanese Interval Walking-Power Meets Precision
In 1996, researchers at Shinshu University in Japan began testing a walking method based on a simple principle:
" Alternate bursts of brisk walking with slower recovery intervals."

The results were startling.
Faster fat loss,
Improved cardiovascular markers,
Increased cognitive clarity,
Strength gains in older populations.

Known as Japanese Interval Walking (JIW), the method is now used across Japan in wellness programs for:
Women over 40 experiencing hormonal shifts,
Seniors recovering from inactivity,
Busy professionals looking for maximum benefit in minimum time.

Key features:

3m inutes of fast-paced walking (70-75% max effort),
3 minutes of slow recovery walking,
Repeated for 30 minutes total,
Combined with controlled breathing and posture awareness.

This pattern boosts VO_2 max, mitochondrial efficiency, and helps regulate insulin and cortisol—— all without needing a gym or equipment.

Why"East Meets East" Works.
On paper, Tai Chi Walking and Japanese Interval Walking seem very different.
But look closer:

Element	Tai Chi Walking	Japanese Interval Walking
Breathwork	Deep & synchronized	Patterned for stamina & focus
Posture	Rooted & vertical	Aligned & dynamic
Mindfulness	Meditative	Focused & present
Flow	Continuous & soft	Rhythmic & alternating
Goal	Restore internal balance	Reignite external performance

When fused together, they become lthe perfect yin-yang walking method. One calms. The other activates. Together, they heal.

The Healing Walk Method Is Born.
By merging:
The mind-body wisdom of Tai Chi,
The physiological precision of Japanese Interval Walking,
The emotional needs of the modern adult.

… we create a method that is:
> Gentle but powerful,
> Rhythmic but purposeful,
> Fat-burning and stress-reducing,
> Accessible yet transformative.

And most importantly: it fits into real life—— no need for studios, mats, or trainers.Just your body, your breath, and the right method.

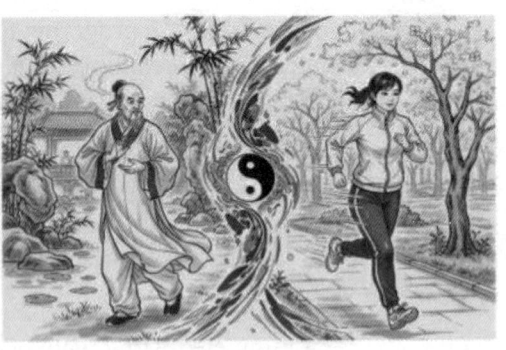

You' re not just borrowing two techniques.You' re stepping into a whole new way of moving—— one that respects where you are today, and leads you exactly where you want to go.

The 3 Core Pillars Of The healing Walk Method.

You now know that simply walking isn't enough—— and that ancient movement traditions offer powerful alternatives. But what exactly makes The healing Walk Method so effective?
It's built on three essential pillars, each one designed to activate a
  different part of your healing system: body, breath, and brain.
Let's explore them one by one.

Pillar 1: Rhythmic Movement.
"When you walk with rhythm, your body remembers how to heal."
This is where form meets function. Unlike casual walking, the healing Walk relies on intentional patterns. You're not just moving—— you're creating internal cadence that:
> Balances your nervous system
> Activates fat- burning through interval bursts
> Enhances circulation, oxygenation, and lymph flow
> Protects joints while building stamina

There are two types of rhythm we focus on:
> 1. Interval Rhythm- Alternating between brisk and slow walking (from JapaneseInterval Walking).
> 2. Fluid Rhythm- Continuous, mindful stepping in alignment with posture (from TaiChi Walking).

When combined, they train your body to move with both efficiency and grace, building endurance without stress or pain.

Pillar 2: Conscious Breathing.
"Your breath is the remote control of your nervous system."
Most people walk while holding their breath unconsciously—or breathing shallowly through the chest. In the healing Walk Method, breathing is not optional—— it's central.
We teach you how to:
> Breathe in through the nose for energy,
> Breathe out through the mouth for release,
> Use breath- to- step ratios (like 3:3 or 4:4) to build endurance,
> Engage diaphragmatic breath for inner calm and organ massage.

This improves:
> Oxygen utilization,
> Mental clarity,
> Emotional regulation,
> Immune strength,

Your breath becomes a metronome that synchronizes your steps with your healing state.

Pillar 3: Mindful Posture.
"How you hold yourself determines how you feel."
Posture isn't just about appearance —— it directly affects your nervous system, digestion, and energy.
With the healing Walk Method, posture becomes an active tool for healing. You'll learn how to:
> Align your head over heart, and heart over pelvis,
> Ground through your feet while lifting through your spine,
> Keep the shoulders open without tension,
> Let your arms swing naturally in coordination with breath,
>
> Keep your gaze soft and forward—— not downward.

This pillar draws heavily from Tai Chi walking mechanics, and builds postural intelligence with each step. No forced tension. No robotic form. Just fluid awareness.

> When All Three Pillars Combine...
> Imagine this:
>> You walk in intervals, switching gears like a wave.
>> Your breath guides the speed and intensity of each step.
>> Your posture supports your organs, your spine, and your confidence.

That's The Healing Walk Method in action.
It's not a workout. It's a living practice —— where each component

reinforces the others to restore rhythm, resilience, and inner calm.

Quick Summary:

Pillar	Focus	Result
Rhythmic Movement	Timing, pattern, intervals	Fat loss, joint health, cardiovascular boost
Conscious Breathing	Breath control & alignment	Stress relief, stamina, focus
Mindful Posture	Alignment & fluidity	Pain relief, confidence, energy balance

With these three pillars, you're no longer walking for fitness.
You're walking to realign your body, calm your mind, and restore your energy at the source.

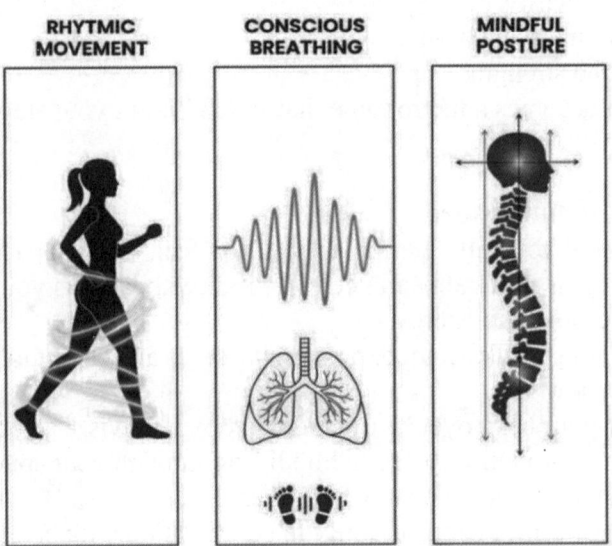

Why This Method Works Especially For Women Over 40

Something begins to shift around age 40.
You start waking up feeling tired even after 8 hours of sleep.
Your body holds onto weight differently—— especially around the belly.
You feel invisible in your own skin, chasing energy that once came easily.
Your works aren't working like they used to.
And worst of all?
You're doing everything "right", yet nothing seems to move.
It's not a willpower problem.
It's a biology problem ——and The Healing Walk Method is built to solve it.

What's Really Going On After 40?
Let's talk about the real culprits——the ones most fitness programs ignore:
  Hormonal fluctuations(estrogen, cortisol, thyroid changes),
  Inflammation and oxidative stress build up silently,
  Sleep quality declines as melatonin production drops,
  Mitochondria(your energy factories) start to slow down,
  Stress tolerance lowers, especially with caregiving or career shifts,
  Blood sugar and insulin become harder to regulate,
  Intense workouts now lead to more fatigue and inflammation, not progress.

This is where traditional fitness fails women over 40. It pushes harder when your body is already overwhelmed. It treats you like a 25-year-old —— instead of the intelligent, evolved, powerful system you are today.

Why The Healing Walk Method Works Now.
Our method speaks the language your body now understands:
  Gentle intensity—— enough to trigger fat loss and muscle tone, without stress,
  Breath control—— lowering cortisol, supporting hormones,
  Rhythmic flow—— rebalancing your nervous system and reducing cravings,
  Joint-friendly movement —— protecting knees, hips, spine,
  Mindfulness —— reconnecting you with your body instead of punishing it,
  Adaptability—— fitting into real life, not demanding rigid routines.

You don't need another challenge.
You need a daily ritual that heals while it reshapes.

The Psychology of Women 40+ — And How We Honor It.
You're not motivated by aesthetics alone.
You're motivated by:
- Feeling strong and self-led again,
- Reclaiming calm, clarity, and balance,
- Having energy for those you love,
- Reversing burnout—— not ignoring it,
- Aging vibrantly, not silently.

The Healing Walk Method is designed around your priorities, not society's outdated ideals. It's not about pushing through pain. It's about partnering with your body, shifting from self-doubt to self-trust—— one rhythmic step at a time.

A Method That Aligns with the Female Body.

Common Issue	Our Method's Solution
Cortisol overload	Breathwork syncs steps with calm
Sluggish metabolism	Interval walking boosts VO_2+ fat burn
Hormonal imbalances	Rhythmic movement supports endocrine balance
Joint stiffness	Tai Chi patterns improve fluid mobility
Mental fog	Focused steps+ breath = cognitive clarity

What Women Say After Trying This Method:
"I feel like my body is finally listening to me."
"I sleep better. I'm calmer. My jeans fit again."
"This is the first time in years I've moved without pain or guilt."
"It's not just walking... it's walking with power and peace."
These aren't side effects.
They're design features —— for you.

This isn't about "bouncing back."
It's about moving forward—— with rhythm, grace, and full-body healing.

CHAPTER 3-GETTING STARTED: YOUR HEALING WALK PLAN

What You Need (And Don't Need) To Begin.
Let's start with a liberating truth:
You don't need fancy gear, a gym, or hours of free time to transform your body and mind. In fact, the more complicated the method, the less likely it is to last.
The Healing Walk Method is designed to be simple, flexible, and low-barrier, especially for people who already carry heavy schedules, emotional fatigue, or physical limitations.
Let's remove the friction and focus on what truly matters.

What You Don't Need:
- × No gym membership,
- × No expensive trackers or fitness apps,
- × No weights, resistance bands, or mats,
- × No "perfect" outfit or shoes,
- × No high-impact movements or choreography,
- × No prior experience with Tai Chi or walking protocols.

Forget the perfection paralysis.
You already have everything you need — starting with your body and breath.

What You Do Need:

Essential	Why It Matters
Comfortable walking shoes	Protect joints, improve rhythm
30 minutes, 4-5x/ week	Sustainable and effective routine
Open space (indoors or outdoors)	Freedom of movement, mental clarity
Willingness to breathe with intention	Activates the healing state
Curiosity to connect with your body	Builds long-term success

Optional (but useful):
- A basic timer or stopwatch,
- A journal to track mood/ energy before and after walks,
- Earbuds with calming music or nature sounds,
- A partner (human or dog!) to walk with for accountability.

Indoor vs. Outdoor: What's Better?
The best environment is the one you'll actually use.
However, we recommend outdoor walking whenever possible because:
- Sunlight helps regulate circadian rhythm and mood,
- Nature exposure lowers cortisol,

Varying terrain naturally engages stabilizer muscles,Open space = open mind.

That said, you can absolutely do this indoors ——in your hallway, around your living room, or even in a small backyard.

The method adapts to your reality, not the other way around.

What If I'm Out of Shape or Injured?

Then you're in the right place.
This method is:
- Low-impact,
- Joint-friendly,
- Scalable (you can shorten duration, slow down intervals, rest more often),
- Designed with neurorehabilitation principles that gently retrain movement and posture without pain.

We'll give you adaptations in Chapter 5, but for now, know this:
If you can breathe and take a few steps, you can begin.

Reframe the Start: It's Not a Workout— It's a ritual.

Your healing walk is not another chore.
It's your daily exhale, your moment of reconnection, your small rebellion against burnout.
So don't overthink it.
Set your shoes by the door.
Pick a time you can repeat.
And just start.

You don't need a new life.
You need a new rhythm——— one step at a time.

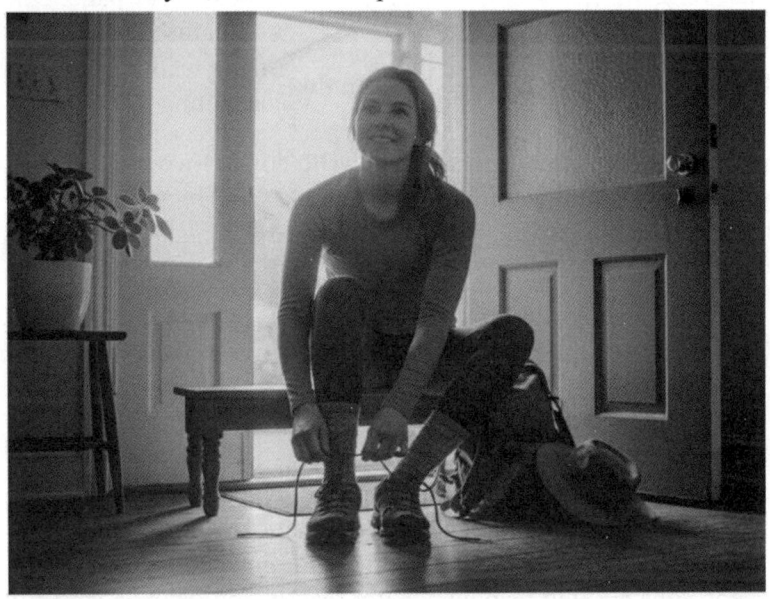

The Optimal Walking Schedule For Healing, Balance, And Energy.

Consistency always beats intensity—— especially after 40.
The Healing Walk Method is not about pushing harder, but walking smarter.
This isn't a traditional "fitness schedule." It's a nervous system healing protocol, designed to work with your body's natural recovery rhythm —— not against it.
Let's break down the weekly schedule that maximizes energy, fat burn, hormone balance, and emotional calm—— with zero crash.

The Healing Walk Weekly Blueprint:

Day	Focus	Time	Notes
Monday	Interval Activation	30 min	3:3 brisk/ slow ratio, start the week energized
Tuesday	Recovery Flow	20-30min	Tai Chi Walking style: slow, mindful, restorative
Wednesday	Power Rhythm	30-35min	Intervals + breath focus (4:4 breathing)
Thursday	Rest or 15 min gentle walk		Optional, restorative only
Friday	Mind-Body Sync	30 min	Mixed intervals + posture awareness
Saturday	Open Walk	25-40min	Choose your pace, connect with nature
Sunday	Integration Day	20-30min	Gentle walking+ reflection journaling

Optional Enhancer: After each session, write down 3 words to describe how you feel. This builds mind-body awareness and shows real-time results beyond calories.

Why Alternating Intensity Works Best After 40.
Alternating days of higher activation with recovery walks is not random —— it's based on:
  Heart Rate Variability (HRV) optimization,
  Cortisol cycle balancing,
  Mitochondrial recovery rhythms,
  Immune modulation: keeping inflammation low.
  Preventing sympathetic dominance (chronic stress response).
This keeps your body in responsive, not reactive mode —— meaning you burn fat without triggering a survival stress state.

Weekly Goals-What to Expect.
By following this rhythm for 2-3 weeks, you can expect:

Result	Why It Happens
✔ Improved sleep	Breath + rhythm calm your nervous system
✔ Reduced cravings	Balanced cortisol and insulin regulation
✔ More stable mood	Breath-driven walks support serotonin
✔ Reduced bloating	Gentle movement activates digestion
✔ Fat loss (esp. around midsection)	Brisk intervals trigger metabolic shift
✔ Increased energy by day 10-14	Mitochondrial recovery kicks in

These are not hopes.
They are common responses from women and men just like you, when the body stops fighting and starts syncing.

Customize If Needed.
If you're:
    Just starting or recovering→begin with 3 days/ week (Mon-Wed-Fri),
    Stressed or sleeping poorly→emphasize flow days (Tue-Sun),
    Already active→ use this as your recovery+ alignment base.
This isn't a rulebook. It's a healing rhythm that adapts to your season of life.

Weekly Planner(Bonus Template Suggestion).
You'll find a fillable weekly planner in the bonus section —— use it to track:
    Start time,
    Duration,
    Mood before/ after,
    Breath pattern used,
    Any discomfort or breakthroughs.
Tracking creates accountability, motivation, and most importantly——
proof that your body is changing.

You don't need to walk harder.
You need to walk with purpose, breath, and rhythm.
And when you do, your body will begin to change—— from the inside out.

Preparing Your Mind: Setting The Intention Before You Step

Every step begins in the mind —— long before your feet move.
What makes The Healing Walk Method different from any "just go walk" program is this: we don't just tell you to move —— we teach you how to show up mentally before each walk begins.
Because when your intention is aligned with your movement, the body doesn't just burn calories...
It begins to heal.
It reclaims rhythm.
It builds trust with itself again.

Why Intention= Amplification
Most people start exercise in a state of:
- Guilt,
- Pressure,
- Shame,
- Comparison,
- Frustration.

That energy follows you into every step.
But when you pause—— even for 60 seconds—— and reframe the experience as healing, your body begins walking in a different nervous system state.
That state is what flips the switch from:

Old Way	Healing Walk Way
"I have to do this"	"I get to reconnect"
"Let's push harder"	"Let's listen deeper"
"Will this burn enough fat?"	"How does my body feel today?"
"I'm behind"	"I'm building forward"

🔥3-Step Pre-Walk Intention Ritual (Takes 2 Minutes or Less).

Step 1: Ground Physically.
Stand tall.
Feet hip-width apart.
Take one slow, deep breath in.
Exhale fully.
Let your shoulders drop.
Feel gravity support your body.
Say quietly (or think):
"This walk is a gift. I'm here."

Step 2: Choose a Micro- Intention.

Ask yourself: "What do I want to feel or release during this walk?"
Choose one word:
- Calm,
- Strength,
- Clarity,
- Energy,
- Gratitude,
- Joy,
- Trust,
- Recovery.

Repeat it mentally on your first few steps—— let it lead you.

Step 3: Smile (Gently).

It may sound silly. But studies show that smiling—— even slightly—— changes your breath and hormone profile instantly.
- Lowers cortisol,
- Boosts dopamine,
- Activates "approach" energy vs. avoidance.

Smile. Even just with your eyes.
Let your system know:
"This is safety. This is care. This is mine."

Why This Mental Prep Changes Everything:

Intention Set	Result
"I choose calm"	Breath deepens faster, pace slows naturally
"I choose strength"	Posture realigns, stride becomes more rooted
"I choose energy"	Brain releases norepinephrine, boosting alertness
"I choose joy"	Natural dopamine increase sustains motivation

This is neurohormonal training—— not fluff.
You're training your nervous system to associate movement with safety, not stress.
Over time, you'll notice:
- You crave walks instead of forcing them,
- You feel more like "you" within the first few steps,
- Your body responds faster—— because it trusts the pattern.

Pro Tip: Anchor Your Intention.
If possible, create a ritual anchor—— something small but repeatable——— that reminds your brain, "we're about to walk and heal."
Examples:
- Touch your heart before you leave
- Look out a window and breathe before lacing shoes
- Light a candle or set a tone on your phone

Use a mantra: "I walk to remember my strength."

Small cues= big neurological trust.

A walk without intention is just motion.
A healing Walk with intention becomes a ritual of recovery.

Walking Into Flow: How To Feel Your Body Instead Of Fighting It.

Most people walk the way they live:
hurried, distracted, and disconnected.
They push through right hips, ignore pain in their knees, or rush to hit a step count ──────── all while staying stuck in their own heads.
But when you walk with awareness, a shift begins.
You enter what neuroscience calls"the flow state"──── and what ancient traditions call"returning home to the body."
This is the foundation of The healing Walk Method.

What Is Flow ────── and Why Does It matter?
Flow is a state where:
      Time slows down
      Self-consciousness fades
      Movement feels effortless
      You' re fully engaged, without force
Healing hormones like dopamine and endorphins naturally riseIt's a neurological sweet spot where your mind, body, and breath are in perfect synchrony.And walking is the most accessible way to access this healing flow.

Flow = Nervous System Reset
Your nervous system has two main settings:

System	Function
Sympathetic (Fight/ Flight)	Stress, reactivity, survival
Parasympathetic (Rest/ Digest/ Heal)	Recovery, regulation, clarity

When you' re always"on," your body can't heal ──── it's too busy defending.
Flow flips the switch toward healing by:
      Slowing your breathing
      Syncing your steps with your heartbeat
      Quieting the mind's overthinking
      Creating sensorimotor integration (body + brain working together)

How to Walk Into Flow-5 Simple Triggers.

1. Start with Sensation.
    Instead of marching, pause and ask:
    "What does my body feel like... right now?"
    Feel the soles of your feet.
    The sway of your arms.
    The weight shift from heel to toe.
    The breath expanding your ribs.
    The more you notice, the faster you enter flow.
2. Use Repetition to Drop In.
    Step. Breathe. Step. Breathe.
    This repetition acts like a meditative rhythm that quiets mental noise.
    Try this sequence:
    3 steps in (inhale through nose).
    3 steps out (exhale through mouth).
    Repeat for 2-3 minutes, then let breath find its natural pace.
    This is called neurological entrainment—— syncing body and breath to rhythm.
3. Shift from Achievement to Awareness.
    Instead of thinking:
    "Am I doing it right?"
    Ask:
    "Can I feel more ease in this moment?"
    Replace:
        "Faster"→with →"Fuller"
        "Farther"→ with→"Deeper"
        "Better"→with→"Truer"
    This shift reduces inner resistance —— a major barrier to flow.

4. Engage All Senses.
    Flow isn't just internal —— it's multi-sensory.
    Try focusing on:
        The sound of your steps,
        The feeling of air on your skin,
        The colors around you (even in grayscale if indoors),
        The rhythm of your breath.
These inputs anchor you into the present moment, which is where healing happens.

5. Allow Emotions to Move
    You might notice feelings rising while walking:
    sadness, frustration, relief, clarity.
    That's not a breakdown—— it's a release.

Walking moves energy. And when you stop fighting your body, your emotional body responds too.
Let it happen. It's part of the flow. It's part of the healing.
Flow= The Healing State.

Old Pattern	Flow State Rewiring
Resistance	Acceptance
Fatigue	Energy
Overthinking	Embodiment
Disconnection	Integration
Stress response	Recovery mode

Every flow-state walk teaches your nervous system that movement is safe.
That your body is a resource, not a burden.
That healing doesn't have to hurt.

You don't need to control your body.
You need to listen to it long enough for it to trust you again.

CHAPTER 4

The Basic healing Walk Sequence (Step- By- Step).

This is not just a walk—— it's a ritual in motion.
In this chapter, you'll learn the core sequence of The healing Walk Method ——a simple yet powerful practice designed to:
- Activate healing physiology,
- Harmonize breath and body,
- Restore natural posture,
- Trigger fat burning without stress,
- Build consistency and trust in movement.

It's ideal for:
- Beginners,
- People in recovery or burnout,
- Women 40+,
- Anyone looking for a calming, fat- burning, healing reset.
- Let's go step- by- step.

🧘 HEALING WALK-FULL SEquence (15-30 MINUTES).

①Grounding(2-3 minutes).
This first step tells your nervous system:
"We' re safe. We' re home. Let's begin."
How:
    1. Stand tall, feet hip-width apart,
    2. Breathe in slowly through the nose(count 4),
    3. Exhale gently through the mouth(count 4),
    4. Let arms hang naturally,
    5. Soften knees slightly,
    6. Feel feet pressing into the ground,
    7. Gently smile.
Repeat 3-5 breaths before starting your first step.

② gentle Start(3 minutes).
Purpose: To wake up body awareness and rhythm.
How:
    Begin walking slowly and silently,
    Focus on the sound of your steps,
    Breathe naturally,
    Let arms swing without tension,
    Stay present in your body.
Try this mantra:
"Every step is healing. Every breath is strength."

③ Rhythm & breath Phase (12-20 minutes).
This is the core of the session—— combining walking pace + breath + mindful presence.
Step Pattern:
    Walk at a moderate pace (brisk but not rushed),
    Count your steps and match them to your breath.
Breath Sync Option 1(standard):
    Inhale for 3 steps,
    Exhale for 3 steps,
    Repeat in a gentle rhythm.
Breath Sync Option 2(advanced/ energy boost):
    Inhale for 4 steps,
    Exhale for 4 steps,
    Add a slight hold after exhale (1 step).
If you lose count, it's okay. Gently return.
The goal isn't perfection —— it's presence.

④Mind-Body Integration (2-3 minutes).
This is your cooldown of awareness —— reconnecting with breath, emotion, and sensation.
How:
> Slow your pace,
> Return to natural breath,
> Observe: What do I feel right now?
> Place one hand on your heart as you stop,
> Close your eyes for a moment,
> Inhale deeply once,
> Exhale slowly.

Whisper (or think):
"Thank you, body. We did this together."

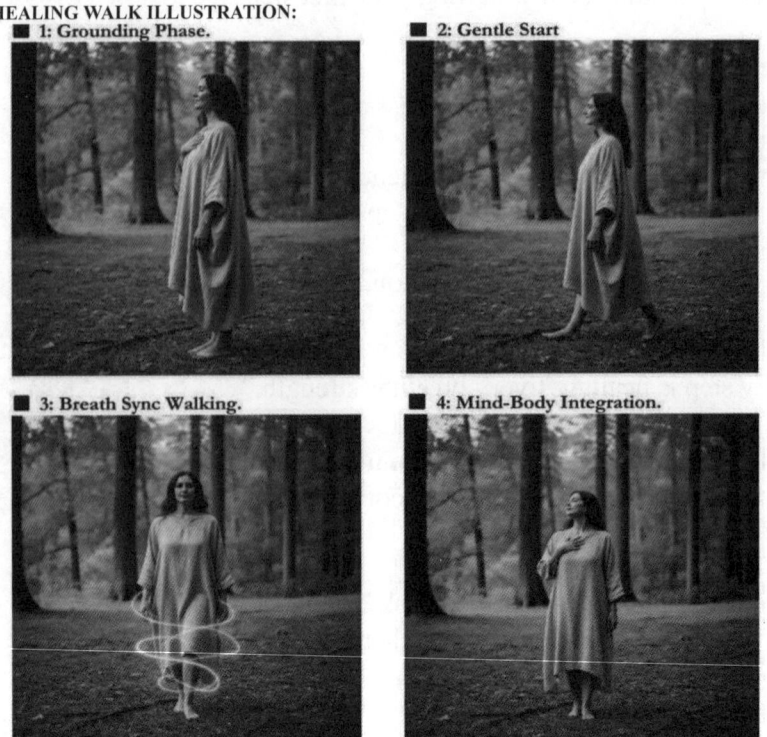

HEALING WALK ILLUSTRATION:
1: Grounding Phase.
2: Gentle Start
3: Breath Sync Walking.
4: Mind-Body Integration.

One walk like this can change your mood. A few can change your energy. But walking like this consistently? That can change your life.

Breathwork Techniques That Unlock Deeper healing.

Breathing is not just survival—— it's the most direct, immediate way to reset your nervous system. Most people breathe like they live: shallow, rushed, and unaware.

But when you walk with conscious breath, you create a flow of oxygen, energy, and calm through every cell of your body.

In The healing Walk Method, breath is not an accessory—— it's a foundational pillar of healing.

🖊 Why Breath matters (Especially After 40)

As we age—— and especially for women in perimenopause and beyond —— breath becomes:

    A hormone stabilizer,

    A mood regulator,

    A fat-burn accelerator,

    A pain reducer,

    A gateway to parasympathetic dominance (the healing state).

Controlled breath = controlled cortisol.

And cortisol is the master switch for belly fat, anxiety, poor sleep, cravings, and chronic fatigue.

3 BREATH TECHNIQUES FOR HEALING WALKS
(You'll learn when and how to use each one)

1. The 3:3 Walking breath.
Use for: Daily walks, rhythm entrainment, mental focus.
How to do it:

>Inhale through the nose for 3 steps,
>Exhale through the mouth for 3 steps,
>Repeat for 3-10 minutes.

This creates rhythm, balances CO_2/O_2, and brings calm alertness
Great for morning or mid- day walksOptional cue mantra:"Balance in. Balance out."

2. The 4:4 Deep healing breath.
Use for: Fatigue, burnout, emotional overwhelm.
How to do it:

>Inhale through the nose for 4 steps,
>Exhale through the mouth for 4 steps,
>Keep pace slow and even,
>Walk gently, feel each footstep.

Triggers vagus nerve for parasympathetic activation,
Supports digestion, sleep, and emotional regulation.
Pro tip: Drop your shoulders each time you exhale.
Optional cue mantra:
" Release. Receive."

3. The 2:6 Detox Breath.
Use for: Stress release, anxiety, inflammation reduction.
How to do it:

>Inhale through the nose for 2 steps,
>Exhale through the mouth for 6 steps,
>Slow your pace to match the breath,
>Keep lips soft and jaw relaxed.

Promotes carbon dioxide clearance.
>✓ Calms hyperactive brain states.
>✓ Helps reduce bloating and water retention.

Optional cue mantra:
"Let it go… all of it."

When to Use Each Breath:

Time of Day	Best Breath Technique
Morning	3:3 Walking Breath
Midday Stress	4:4 Deep Healing
Evening Wind-Down	2:6 Detox
Post-Meal Bloat	2:6 Detox
Emotional Upset	4:4 or 2:6
High Energy Day	3:3 Walking

Match your breath to your intention, not your clock.

The Science Behind It (Explained Simply).
When you match your steps to breath:

> Your nervous system synchronizes,
> Your heart rate stabilizes,
> Your brain releases alpha waves→ linked to calm focus,
> You burn fat more efficiently (especially with longer exhales),
> You build neural pathways of peace, not panic.

This is not new-age fluff.
It's somatic self-regulation backed by biomechanics and neuroscience.

Tips for Success.
> Start slow —— it's normal to lose count,
> Use headphones with breath-paced soundtracks (bonus provided),
> Don't over-control —— let rhythm guide you,
> Smile lightly —— it unlocks deeper breath.

1-Breath Sync Steps(3:3).

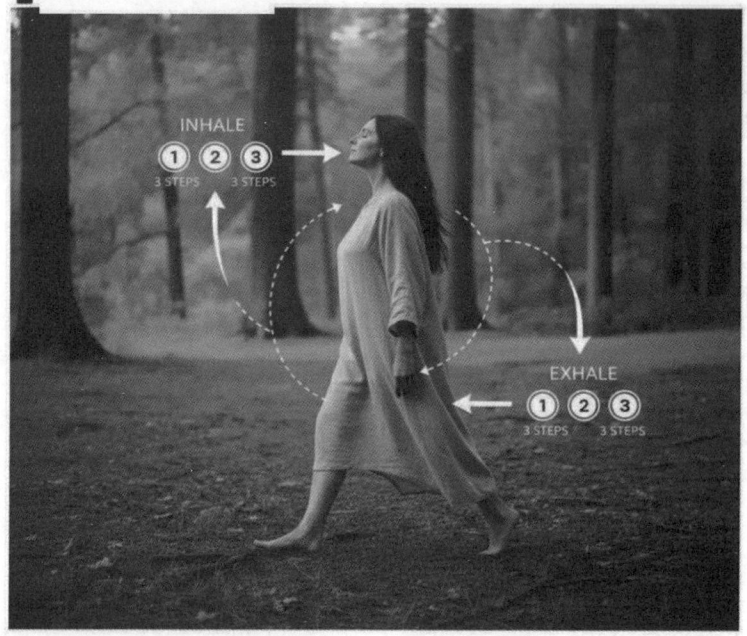

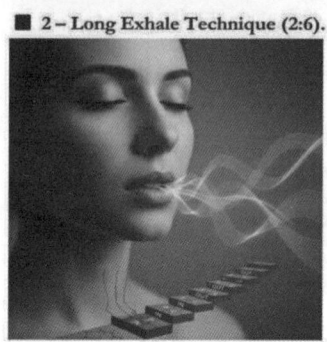

2 – Long Exhale Technique (2:6).

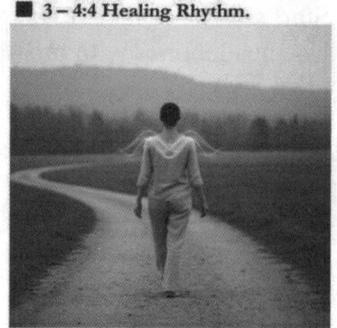

3 – 4:4 Healing Rhythm.

You don't need a new diet.
You don't need another pill.
You need to walk and breathe like your body was always meant to.

Posture Reset: Aligning Your Body For Long- TermMobility & Grace.

Healing begins when the body realigns—— not with effort, but with awareness.
If you' ve ever felt:
    Neck or shoulder pain during walks,
    Tight hips or lower back aches after standing,
    "Hunched" posture in photos,
    Less graceful than you used to be...
You' re not broken.

Your posture needs to be reminded how to hold you—— not punished into submission.
The healing Walk Method resets posture through soft repetition, neural activation, and walking-based alignment.

Why Posture is Nervous System Feedback.
Posture isn't just physical—— it's emotional and neurological.
When you walk compressed, your brain receives signals of:
    Stress,
    Lack of safety,
    Aging,
    Inflammation,
    Exhaustion.
When you walk aligned, your body tells the brain:"We are stable. We are s trong. We are present."

The 5- Point Posture Reset (While Walking).
No mirror. No tension. Just these 5 cues—— done gently while walking.
1. Crown Lifted.
    Imagine a string pulling the top of your head upward—— not forward.
    Chin level to the ground
    Neck long
    Avoid looking down unless needed
    Cue:"at your crown like a queen."
2. Shoulders Melted.
    Let your shoulders slide down and back, not forced—— just released.
    Open chest without puffing
    Arms swing from relaxed shoulders
    Cue:"Let your shoulders drip away from your ears."
3. Core Lightly Engaged.

No squeezing: Just a gentle lift of your lower belly.
Feel your lower abs supporting the pelvis
Avoid arching your back
Cue:"Lift your center like holding a warm bowl inside."

4. Pelvis Neutral.
Think of your hips like a bowl of water—— don't spill it forward or backward.
Don't tuck under,
Don't stick out,
Just let it rest.
Cue:" Balance the bowl."

5. feet Straight, Soft Landing.
Feet point forward, not out like a duck.
Land heel to toe,
Keep knees slightly soft,
Feel each step——— don't slap the ground.
Cue:" Step into softness, not into the fight."

The Walking Alignment Reset (Practice).
Try this 3-minute drill at the start of your walk:
1. Stop. Stand still.
2. Breathe in (4 counts)— crown up.
3. Breathe out(4 counts)— shoulders melt.
4. Breathe in— engage low belly.
5. Breathe out— balance pelvis.
6. Start walking slowly.
7. Step… feel your feet.
8. Adjust gently, one cue at a time.

Do this daily for 2 weeks and observe how your:
Back pain reduces,
Breath gets deeper,
Steps feel more confident,
Walk becomes more graceful and youthful.

Posture Reframe:

Old Belief	Healing Walk Reframe
"My posture is bad"	"My body forgot —— now it remembers"
"I'm getting stiff"	"I'm softening back into mobility"
"I look older"	"I move like I care for myself"

You don't need discipline.
You need reminders—— loving, somatic, consistent.

■ 1 – 5-Point Posture Summary Diagram.   ■ 2 – Before vs. After Posture (Side View).

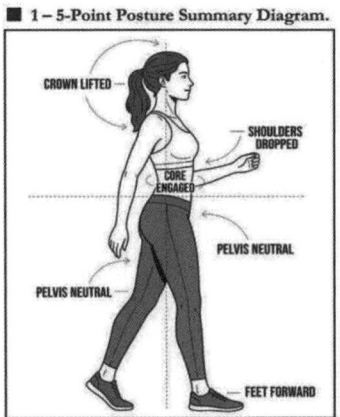
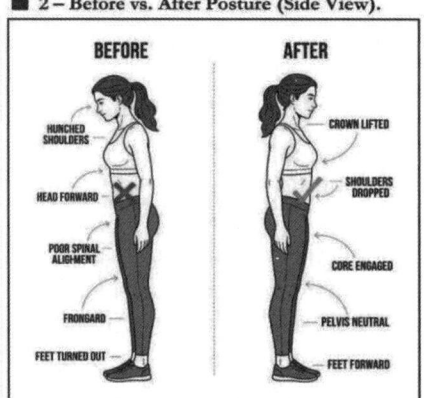

■ 3 – Emotional Posture Shift.

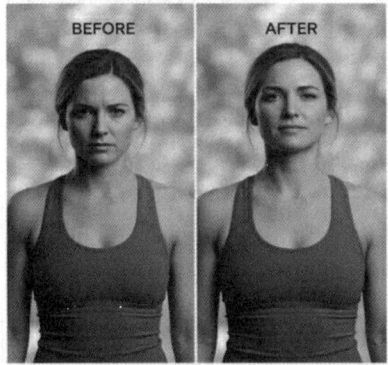

Don't force perfect posture.
Walk gently into alignment—— and your body will remember how to hold you with love.

THE WALKING FLOW PROTOCOL
(Your Daily 15-30 Minute Template for Healing and Energy)

"I want to walk, but I don't know where to start."
"I never stick with routines."
"I need something simple —— but that actually works."
That's exactly what this section is for.
You don't need a complicated plan.
You don't need 10,000 steps.
You need a simple daily rhythm that:
- ✓ Regulates your emotions,
- ✓ Rebalances your hormones,
- ✓ Restores energy,
- ✓ Relieves stiffness,
- ✓ Feels like self-love, not punishment.

The Healing Walk Protocol.
One framework. Two versions. Infinite transformation.

Option A-15-Minute Reset (Short & Powerful).
Perfect for:
- Busy mornings,
- Office breaks,
- Low-energy days,
- Bad weather(can be done indoors).

Step-by-step template:

Time	Phase	Instructions
2min	Grounding	Stand still, breathe 4-4, soften body
3min	Body Awareness Walk	Walk slowly, feel feet, sync breath 3:3
5min	Flow Rhythm Walk	Increase pace slightly, continue 3:3 or 4:4
3min	Integration	Slow down, return to natural breath, gratitude

Cue mantra: "I return to myself with each step."

Option B-30-Minute Transformation Walk.
Perfect for:
- Morning energy boost,
- Stress or anxiety reset,
- Evening decompression,
- Weight loss & fat burn support.

Step-by-step template:

Time	Phase	Instructions
3min	Stillness Grounding	Breath sync (4:4), gentle posture reset
5min	Sensorial Awakening	Walk slowly, focus on breath, feet, wind
10 min	Core Flow	Walk at moderate pace, breath 3:3 or 4:4
5min	Optional Add-On	Try Japanese Intervals or Tai Chi Walking steps
5min	Soft Landing	Cool down walk, smile gently, hand on heart
2min	Stillness Again	Eyes closed, deep exhale, gratitude phrase

Cue mantra:"I am not rushing toward life——I am walking with it."

Real Life = Real Flexibility
Modify daily based on:

If You Feel…	Try This
Tired or sore	15-min reset with breath 4:4
Energetic	30-min full protocol+ intervals
Stressed	Walk slowly with 2:6 detox breath
Bloated or heavy	30-min with long exhales + upright posture
Sad	Walk gently, focus on feet and heart space
Rushed	Do 5 minutes grounding only—— still counts!

Weekly Healing Walk Flow:

Day	Walk Type	Duration	Focus
Monday	Reset	15 min	Re-center body & breath
Tuesday	Core Flow	30 min	Energy & hormone boost
Wednesday	Mindful Short	15 min	Emotional check-in
Thursday	Interval + Flow	30 min	Fat burn & mobility
Friday	Healing Grace	15 min	Walk + posture alignment
Saturday	Full Practice	30+ min	Flow, breath, gratitude
Sunday	Still Walk	10-20 min	Peace, nature, silence

=The Science of Repetition.
The body learns through movement. The mind learns through rhythm.
The heart heals through presence. This isn't a workout plan.
It's a neuro-somatic retraining method disguised as a walk.
You don't need to walk for hours.
You need to walk with intention —— even for 15 minutes.
And repeat it. Until your body remembers...
"This is who I am no

CHAPTER 5: JAPANESE INTERVAL WALKING & CORE TAI CHI FORM

What It Is And Why It Works

Not all intervals are created equal.
This one is backed by science and simplicity.
Japanese Interval Walking (JIW) is a rhythmic method developed by researchers at ShinshuUniversity in Japan.

It's based on short bursts of faster walking alternated with recovery phases, using a very simple formula:
    3 minutes of fast- paced walking,
    3 minutes of slower walking,
    Repeat for 5 sets = 30 minutes total.

This sequence has been clinically shown to improve:
    Cardiovascular health,
    VO_2 max (oxygen use),
    Insulin sensitivity,
    Waist circumference,
    Muscle strength,
    Fat oxidation.

And unlike traditional HIIT?
It doesn't exhaust you. It revives you.
Clinical Results That matter.

Here's what researchers found after 5 months of Japanese Interval Walking in adults aged 45-75:
    10% improvement in aerobic capacity
    12% drop in blood pressure
    6% drop in body fat
    15% improvement in leg muscle strength

Participants also reported:
    Better mood,
    Improved sleep,
    Stronger sense of physical confidence,
    Less joint discomfort.

And most importantly?
They stuck with it.

Why It Works Especially Well for Women 40+
As women age, they face:
- Estrogen drop→affects energy, mood, metabolism.
- Muscle loss→makes walking feel harder.
- Fat retention in belly & hips.
- Hormonal weight resistance (stress = cortisol = stubborn fat).

Japanese Interval Walking solves this by:
- Giving a fat-burning push without long duration,
- Releasing dopamine & endorphins,
- Supporting joint function,
- Resetting cortisol naturally,
- Offering visible progress →motivation.

The Neurometabolic Effect.
The alternation of pace creates a dopamine loop:
1. Effort (fast phase) → challenge + engagement
2. Recovery (slow phase) → safety + reward
3. Repetition→progress+ neuroplasticity

This loop rewires motivation and consistency, and that's exactly what our reader needs.
It's not about pushing harder.
It's about moving smarter.
With just 30 minutes a day, your body learns a new story:"I am capable. I am light. I am strong again."

How To Practice Japanese Interval Walking

This is where the transformation becomes real.
No apps. No gym. No guesswork.
Just you, your breath, your legs, and a short walk that rewires your body.

The Simple Rule.
Japanese Interval Walking (JIW) is based on a 6-minute cycle:
- 3 minutes of brisk walking (you feel your breatb rise),
- 3 minutes of slow walking (you recover and reset).
- Repeat that cycle 5 times.
- Total time:30 minutes.
- Frequency:3-4 days a week.

How Fast Is"Brisk"?
Here's a simple test:

During brisk walk: You can talk, but not sing.
During slow walk: You can breathe through your nose easily.

You should feel slightly breathy, heart rate mildly elevated, but never uncomfortable or straining.
If you use a smartwatch or fitness tracker, aim for:
- Brisk: 5.5-6.5km/h (3.4-4.0 mph)
- Slow: 3.0-4.0km/h (1.8-2.5mph)

Your First 14-Day Japanese Walking Plan.
Let's make it brain-proof, stress-free, and instantly doable.

Week 1

Day	Type	Notes
Mon	3 cycles (18 min)	Try it indoors or in your street
Tue	Rest or slow walk	Breathe, feel your body
Wed	4 cycles (24 min)	Focus on posture
Thu	Rest or light Tai Chi walk	Blend methods
Fri	5 cycles (30 min)	Full JIW walk
Sat	Bonus: Healing Walk reset	Gratitude + slow rhythm
Sun	Optional JIW (3 cycles)	Or mindful breath walk

Week 2

Day	Type	Notes
Mon	Full JIW (30 min)	Match with 3:3 breath
Tue	Light day	Stillness or 4:4 walk
Wed	Full JIW + bonus Tai Chi step	Flow & strength
Thu	Core Flow Healing Walk	Emotional focus
Fri	Full JIW (focus on breath)	Deeper fat burn
Sat	Nature-based walk	Outdoors, sensory
Sun	Reflection walk	Think about how you feel now vs. before

Pro Tips for Success:
- Set a timer for each 3-minute phase.
- Use playlists with alternating rhythm songs.
- Optional: Use walking apps with interval times.
- Combine with breath patterns (from Chapter 4.2).
- Track your walks in a small notebook or digital log.
- Reward yourself with a self-care ritual after each session.

Customize It for YOUR Life:

If You Feel...	Modify Like This
Too tired	Do 2 cycles only
Anxious	Extend slow phases
High energy	Add a 6th cycle
Need focus	Use breath cue: "Strong-Calm"
Low motivation	Walk with music or audiobooks

Optional Mind- Body Add- Ons
 During slow phase: Add affirmations like:
"I am healing with every step.", "My energy is rising."
During brisk phase: Focus on: "I walk toward strength.",
"Every step burns what I don't need."

How Fast Should I Walk Guide.

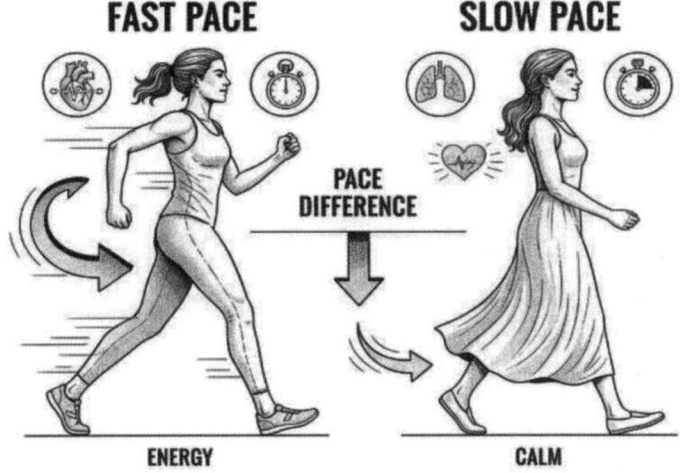

Tracker Template.

MONTHLY CYCLE TRACKER

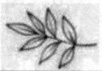

DATE	CYCLES DONE	NOTES

No more waiting to feel better.
Start walking the version of you that's already in motion.
All it takes is 30 minutes——3 times a week—— with intention.

THE CORE TAI CHI WALKING FORM

Step-By-Step Breakdown (Complete Guide)

Tai Chi Walking is not just "slow walking." It is a precise, fluid, mindful movement system that cultivates balance, inner stillness, and flow of energy ("Qi") through the entire body.

Here is the Core Walking Form in a complete step-by-step structure you can learn and repeat, even daily.

STRUCTURE OVERVIEW: 5 ELEMENTS.
1. Starting Posture (Wu Ji).
2. Weight Shifting.
3. Rooting & Stepping.
4. Arm Flow.
5. Breath Synchronization.

STEP-BY-STEP WALKING FORM:

1. Starting Posture-Wu Ji Position.
   - Stand tall, feet shoulder-width apart.
   - Knees soft, pelvis slightly tucked.
   - Spine straight, chin slightly tucked.
   - Shoulders relaxed, arms hanging naturally.
   - Eyes softly gazing forward.
   - Begin with 3 slow deep breaths.

Intention: Let go of tension. "Stand like a mountain, calm like water."

2. Weight Shifting-Feel the Root.
   - Shift your body weight fully onto your right foot.
   - Left foot becomes "empty"——— light, floating.
   - Pause and feel grounded in your standing leg.
   - Shift back to center, then to left.

This phase awakens body awareness and balance.

3. Rooting & Stepping-The Tai Chi Step.
   1. From your weighted right leg, slowly peel off the left heel.
   2. Let toes remain in contact a moment——— then lift gently.
   3. Move left foot forward (6-8 inches)——— keep it low, almost brushing the ground.
   4. Touch heel first——— softly——— then roll the foot flat.
   5. Shift your weight slowly forward into the new leg.
   6. Repeat on the opposite side.

Focus: One step at a time. Each movement is a circle, not a line.

4. Arm Flow-Natural Spiral Movement.

- As you step forward with the left foot:
  ○ The right arm rises forward (as if pushing clouds),
  ○ The left arm lowers softly to the side.
- Arms follow a gentle curve————— never stiff.
- When you step with the right foot, reverse the motion.

Imagine moving underwater: arms glide, not swing.
Each step= breath = spiral.

5. Breath Synchronization-The Inner Flow.
   Inhale as you shift weight.
   Exhale as you step forward.
   Or try: Inhale 3 steps/ Exhale 3 steps—— stay rhythmic.
Never hold your breath. Keep the breath circular and soft.

RECOMMENDED PRACTICE SEQUENCE:

Duration	What to Do
2min	Standing posture (Wu Ji) +3 deep breaths
5m in	Weight shifting practice
10 min	Walking form-20 to 30 slow steps
3m in	Standing still to integrate (no movement)

INTENTION DURING WALK:
   "I walk as if kissing the Eartb with my feet."
   "Eacb step is a breatb, each breath is a step."
   "I move with power and softness."

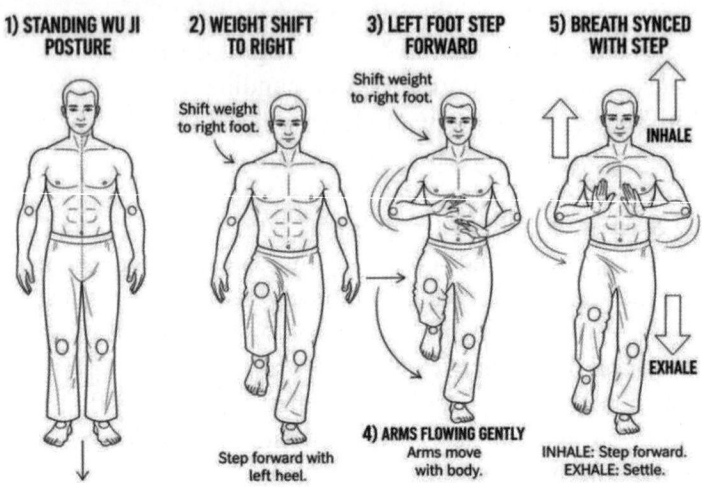

COMMON MISTAKES TO AVOID
During Tai Chi Walking Practice.

An authentic and effective Tai Chi Walking practice is Subtle yet powerful. But it's also easy to unknowingly introduce habits that block energy flow, reduce benefits, or even cause strain over time.

Below, you'll find the most frequent mistakes, along with clear corrections to help you maintain a clean, healing, and safe practice.

1. Moving Too Fast.
    Mistake: Rushing through steps or trying to " walk normally but slower."Fix: Remember: this is not about speed—— it's about awareness. Count your steps. Use breath to slow down. Visualize moving through water.

2. Locking the Knees.
    Mistake: Straightening and locking the knees during or after steps.Fix: Keep knees softly bent. Micro-bending allows energy to pass through the joints and prevents shock or tension buildup.

3. Leaning Forward or Back.
    Mistake: Leaning the upper body to " follow" the foot or "lead" the step.Fix: Imagine a string pulling you upward from the crown of your head. Your spine should stay vertical—— no tilt. Let the legs do the movement, not your torso.

4. Over-swinging the Arms.
    Mistake: Arms flailing, moving stiffly, or swinging like in regular walking.Fix: Tai Chi arms float and spiral. Keep elbows soft. Let the motion be generated by the waist and flow outward. Less is more.

5. Stepping Heel-First Too Aggressively.
    Mistake: Slamming the heel into the ground. Fix: Let the foot kiss the earth. Heel touches first, yes, but gently. Then roll through the foot softly to avoid jarring the knees and hips.

6. Holding the breath.
    Mistake: Forgetting to breathe or breathing shallowly. Fix: Inhale through the nose, exhale softly through the mouth or nose. Match your breath to your step. Stay fluid and full.

7. Thinking Instead of Feeling.
   Mistake: Overanalyzing every move, getting caught in "Is this right?"Fix: Trust your body. Let it learn through repetition. Feel your feet, breath, and flow.Perfection is not the goal——presence is.

PRO TIP:"90% Awareness, 10% Mechanics".
The essence of Tai Chi Walking is internal awareness.
Even if your posture isn't perfect, if your mind is calm, breath flowing, and intention present…you' re already practicing the real thing.

Modifications For Different Ages & Body Types.

Walking Reset is designed to be accessible, but every body is different—
— and personalization increases results, comfort, and safety.

This section provides custom adaptations for:
Different age groups (Young Adults,40+,60+,75+),
Various body types(slim, muscular, curvy, overweight, limited mobility),
Common physical considerations(knee pain, back stiffness, fatigue, balance issues).

These modifications are especially important for long- term adherence, and to ensure everyone can benefit from Tai Chi Walking and Japanese Interval Walking (JIW).

YOUNG ADULTS(18-39):
Goal: Channel energy, manage stress, and build healthy habits.
✔ Use faster interval ratios(20/10 or 30/15).
✔ Sync walk posture early to prevent bad habits.

✔ Avoid rushing through Tai Chi segments— cultivate patience.

40+TO 60+
Goal: Balance stress, energy, and beginning signs of joint discomfort.
✔ Choose moderate intervals(15/15),20-30 mins daily.
✔ Incorporate Tai Chi warm- ups before each walk to loosen hips and spine.
✔ Add Qigong arm swings to improve upper body circulation.
✔ Mind the breath:3-in /3-out cadence is ideal.

60+TO 75+
Goal: Maintain mobility, stability, and emotional clarity.
✔ Prioritize soft, even terrain— avoid pavement.
✔ Extend warm- up phase:5 mins Tai Chi,5 mins slow walking.
✔ Use support if needed (e. g. walking stick with ergonomic grip).
✔ Alternate days with chair Qigong or standing breathwork.

75+ OR LIMITED MOBILITY
Goal: Encourage circulation, confidence, and mental sharpness.

✔ Begin with chair-based Tai Chi or breath exercises.

✔ Walk indoors along hallways if balance is a concern.
✔ Use gentle music to cue rhythm and step.
✔ Work with a partner or caregiver if available.

CURVY / PLUS-SIZE BODIES
✔ Focus on joint alignment: feet under hips, knees soft.
✔ Choose cushioned shoes or barefoot on grass.
✔ Shorter intervals(10/10) avoid strain.
✔ Add Qigong side sways to support lower back.

MUSCULAR /ATHLETIC BUILDS
Tai Chi walking helps release over-contracted muscles.
Use walking to increase parasympathetic recovery(rest & digest).
Add light ankle weights only if posture is excellent.
Avoid competitive mindset— focus on flow, not force.

COMMON PHYSICAL NEEDS & TIPS.

Issue	Modification
Knee pain	Shorten stride; walk slower; avoid incline
Lower back stiffness	Swing arms softly; activate glutes intentionally
Fatigue	Break walks into 2x10min daily
Balance issues	Walk next to a wall/ fence or with a stick
Foot sensitivity	Use soft sandals or go barefoot on grass

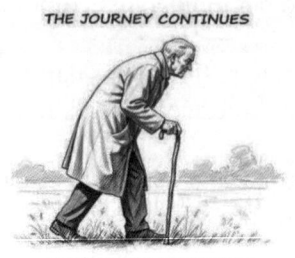

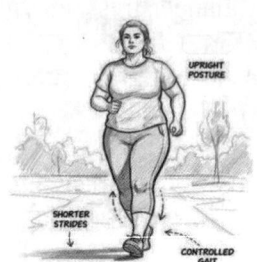

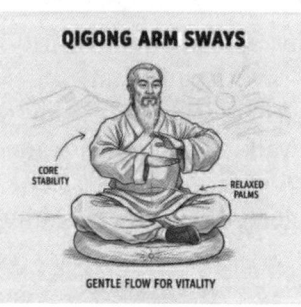

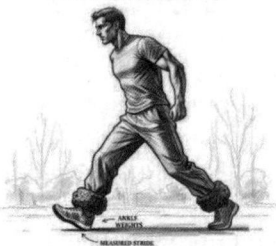

CHAPTER 6: SUGGESTED ROUTINES

Tai Chi Walking+ Japanese Interval Walking (Jiw) Combinations
1).15/15 FUSION ROUTINE:
15 min Tai Chi Walking+15 min Japanese Interval Walking

✦Who it's for: Adults 40+, stressed professionals, beginners transitioning into fitness.

✦How it works: Begin with 15 minutes of slow, mindful Tai Chi Walking (can be static or dynamic).

Follow with 5 rounds of 3- min JIW cycles:
2 mins fast pace (6-7/10 effort)
1 min slow pace (recovery)
Finish with 2-3 mins of Qigong breathing or standing still

✦Goal: Deep reset+ cardiovascular boost without fatigue

2).10/10/10 TRIPLE ROUTINE:
10 min Tai Chi+10 min JIW+10 min Qigong Walking

✦Who it's for: Holistic health seekers, older adults, recovery phase, burnout preventionHow it works:

Tai Chi Walking (10 min): Focus on breath and alignment
JIW(10 min): 3-4 cycles of intervals (2 fast/1 slow)
Qigong Walking(10 min): Use arm sways, relaxed breathing, and intention

✦Goal: Balance Yang (activation) and Yin (recovery). Perfect for daily reset.

3). ALTERNATING DAYS METHOD:
Day 1: Tai Chi Walking+ Qigong
Day 2: JIW + Recovery Stretches
Day 3: Rest or Light Breathing Walk
Repeat

Who it's for: People managing joint pain, low energy, or irregular schedules
How it works:

Cycle energy across the week
No overloading of nervous system or muscles
You stay engaged, recovered, and consistent
Goal: Sustainable transformation- physically, mentally, emotionally.
PRO TIP: Anchor routines to your natural energy rhythm
Morning = JIW or 10/10/10
Midday = Short Tai Chi reset
Evening = Tai Chi+ Qigong combo to unwind

Emotional Awareness Through Each Step.
Walking to Come Back to Yourself

You don't need to fix your emotions.
You need to feel safe enough to feel them.
Emotions Live in the Body—— Not Just the Mind.
We've been taught to sit still when we feel sad, anxious, overwhelmed. But the body remembers everything, and movement is the language it understands.
That's why mindful walking is a somatic (body- based) tool that:
    Releases trapped emotion.
    Regulates nervous system patterns.
    Create s a safe space to feel without being overwhelmed.
    Rebuilds connection between your inner world and outer reality.
This isn't just about walking.
It's about walking yourself back home.

3 Types of Emotional Walking Practices.
Each one is designed to meet you where you are emotionally, with a simple shift in pace, attention, and intention.

1. Calm Walk (For Anxiety, Overthinking)
    Walk pace: Slow, soft
    Focus: Footsteps + nose breathing (4 in / 6 out)
    Cue: "I am safe. This moment is enough."
    Duration: 10-15 minutes
    Optional: Use calming instrumental music
    Do this before sleep or during emotional overload.
2. Fire Walk (For Sadness, Stuck Energy)
    Walk pace: Moderate to brisk
    Focus: belly breath + step rhythm
    Cue: "I am moving forward, even now."
    Duration: 20-25 minutes
    Optional: Walk somewhere symbolic (bridge, nature path)
    Helps shift grief, numbness, or depressive states into motion.
3. Flow Walk (For Reconnection, Presence)
    Walk pace: Natural, playful
    Focus: Alternating senses- what you see, hear, feel
    Cue: "I am in my body. I am in my life."
    Duration: 15-30 minutes
    Optional: Smile slightly while walking
Best when you feel disconnected, "floating," or stuck in your head.

Emotional Check-In: Before You Walk.
Before choosing your walk, ask:
1. What am I feeling right now (without judgment)?
2. Where do I feel it in my body?
3. What kind of walk would help me hold it—— not hide it?

Let the answer guide your steps.

Optional Practice: Walking Emotional Journal.
After your walk, write:
"Today I walked with _____."(emotion)
"It felt like _____ in my body."
"Now I feel _____."

This turns walking into emotional processing, not just exercise.

Lisa's Flow Walk.
Lisa,47, said she felt numb for weeks after burnout. She tried the Flow Walk with the mantra"Iam allowed to enjoy my body."
After a week, she noticed color returning to her thoughts.
"I'm not 'back to normal'—— but I'm no longer frozen," she said.

Calm Walk.   Fire Walk.

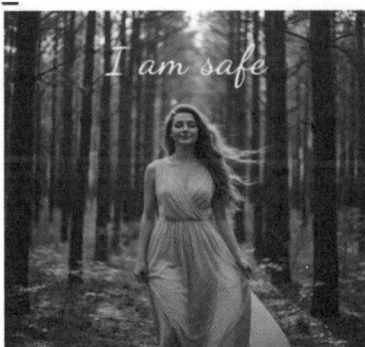 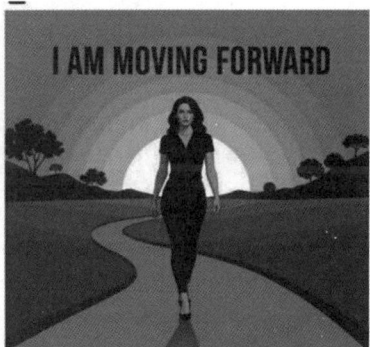

You don't have to"do" anything with your feelings.You just have to walk with them— until they become lighter.

Breath-Based Emotional Detox.

Walking to Breathe Out What No Longer Serves You
When your thoughts won't slow down...
When your chest feels tight...
When your emotions feel stuck...
Breathe with your feet.
Why Breath + Walking Is a Nervous System Reset
Your breath is the remote control of your emotions.
And when you sync your steps with your inhales and exhales, something magical happens:
> Your heart rate synchronizes,
> Your mind slows down,
> Your cortisol drops,
> You stop being reactive,
> You start feeling safe inside,

This is not just relaxation.
It's emotional detox through motion.
Breath Ratios: The Secret Sauce.
Walking with breath ratios is like setting the tempo of your nervous system.
Here are the main breath rhythms we'll use:

Breath Pattern	Emotion It Targets	Best Time To Use
3:3 (inhale 3 steps, exhale 3 steps)	Grounding	Start of walk, stress reset
4:4	Calm focus	Flow walks, morning
4:6	Anxiety, overwhelm	Night, emotional detox
2:6	Rage, agitation	When triggered or tense
6:6	Emotional reconnection	Deep stillness walks

Breathwalk Protocols by Emotion:
For Anxiety or Overthinking:
Breath Pattern:4:6
> Inhale for 4 steps.
> Exhale for 6 steps.
> Walk slowly, eyes soft.
> Cue:"Exbale the noise. Inbale peace.".

Works well in evening or before sleep.
For Anger or Tension:
Breath Pattern:2:6
> Inhale for 2 steps (through nose)
> Exhale for 6 steps (through mouth, slowly)
> Walk with strong steps

Cue:"Release the fire. Ground the body."
Use when agitated or stuck in arguments.

For Sadness or Grief:
Breath Pattern:3:3 or 4:4
- Inhale and exhale equally.
- Walk naturally.
- Cue:"I walk with this feeling. I let it flow.".

Use outdoors, near nature or water if possible.

For Clarity and Centering:
Breath Pattern:6:6
- Long inhales+ long exhales.
- Sync with steps.
- Cue:"I am in my body. I trust this pace.".

Best when you feel"spaced out" or disconnected.

Your 7-Day Breathwalk Reset Plan.

Day	Focus Emotion	Breath Ratio	Duration
Mon	Stress	4:6	15 min
Tue	Focus	4:4	10 min
Wed	Frustration	2:6	20 min
Thu	Sadness	3:3	15 min
Fri	Anxiety	4:6	20 min
Sat	Grounding	6:6	25 min
Sun	Flow+ Joy	Natural breath	30 min

Tips for Mastering Breathwalk:
- Start walking before adjusting breath.
- Walk in silence or with ambient sound.
- Visualize breath as waves under your feet.
- Whisper your mantra to yourself.
- Optional: place hand on heart during slow phases.

Breath Ratios Visualization.

BREATH RATIOS

4:4 EQUAL BREATH

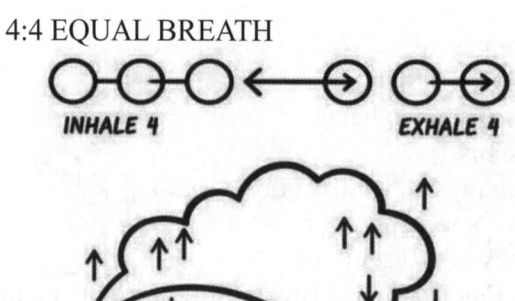

2:6 CALMING BREATH

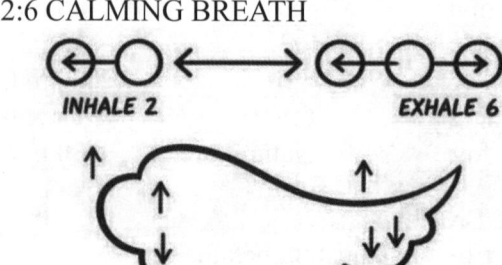

Breathwalk Emotions Map.

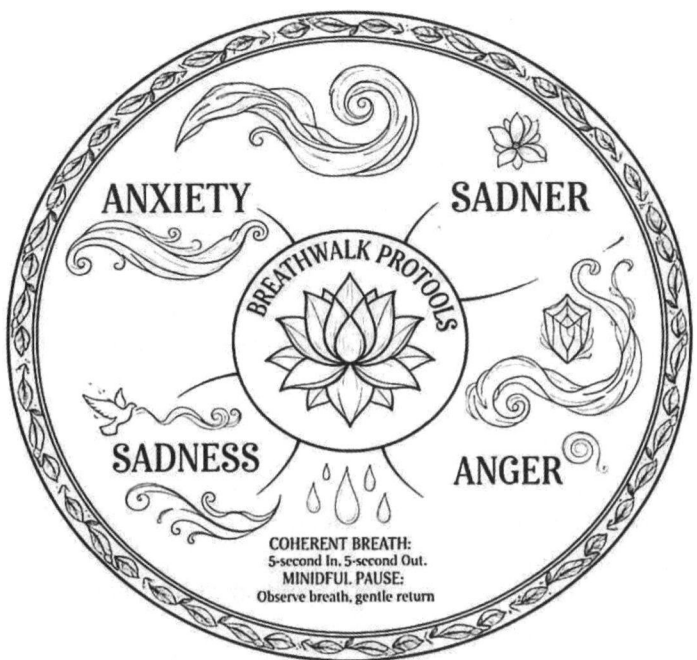

Every emotion has a rhythm.
When you breathe through your feet, you stop drowning in your head.
Walking+ Breath= Emotional sovereignty.

CHAPTER 7: THE INTEGRATIVE RESET.

One week.
Just your feet. Just your breath. Just your presence.
A new you, already waiting.

How This Reset Works.

This 7- day walking reset is designed for:
- Emotional rebalancing,
- Boosting metabolism & energy,
- Reconnecting to your body and motivation,
- Lowering anxiety & mental fog,
- Strengthening walking habit for long- term success.

Each day has:
- A clear intention.
- A physical + emotional focus.
- The specific type of walk to do.
- Optional tools to amplify the effect.
- A simple journal cue.

Let's reset your nervous system, energy, and spirit—— step by step.

DAY 1- Grounding Your Energy.
Type: Tai Chi Walking
Duration: 10-15 min slow pace
Breath Pattern: 3:3
Cue: "I arrive here."
- Focus on your feet touching the ground.
- Visualize releasing tension into the earth.
- Walk with your eyes softly forward.

Journal Prompt:
" Right now, I feel ____ in my body."

DAY 2- Igniting Your Metabolism.
Type: Japanese Interval Walking (3 cycles)
Duration: 18 min
Breath Pattern: Free breathing
Cue: "I am awakening."
- Alternate brisk/ slow every 3 min.
- Swing arms naturally.
- Stand tall, feel strength in legs.

Journal Prompt:
"I felt most alive during ____ ."

DAY3- Clearing Mental Fog.
Type: Flow Walk
Duration: 20-25 min
Breath Pattern: 4:4
Cue: "I let the noise go."
    Switch attention between senses.
    Name things you see, hear, feel.
    Walk with open attention.
Journal Prompt:
"I noticed _____ that I'd been ignoring."

DAY4- Releasing Emotional Tension.
Type: Breathwalk (2:6)
Duration: 20 min
Cue: "I release the fire."
    Walk with firm steps, slow exhales.
    Use whispered mantra.
    Add light shoulder movements.
Journal Prompt:
"Today I let go of _____ ."

DAY5- Building Inner Strength.
Type: Full JIW (5 cycles)
Duration: 30 min
Breath Pattern: Natural
Cue: "I am becoming stronger."
    Embrace the effort.
    Listen to music or silence.
    Count your breaths if distracted.
Journal Prompt:
"I am proud that I _____ ."

DAY6- healing Walk.
Type: Mindful Walk(Flow or Calm)
Duration: 25 min
Breath Pattern: 4:6
Cue: "I walk with compassion."
    Walk near trees, water, or in open space.
    Gentle movements of hands or head.
    Smile slightly, relax jaw.
Journal Prompt:
"I showed myself love by _____ ."

DAY 7- Integration + Gratitude.

Type: Fusion Walk (Free choice of method)
Duration: 20-30 min
Breath Pattern: Your own
Cue:" This is who I am now."
    Mix Tai Chi steps with brisk intervals.
    Pause during the walk to reflect.
    Feel gratitude for what's shifted.
Journal Prompt:
"This week taught me _____."

Optional Enhancements Each Day:
    Ambient playlist with binaural tones.
    Affirmations whispered with breath.
    Take 1 photo after each walk to track progress.
    Use the Daily Reset Log (see bonus) to reflect.

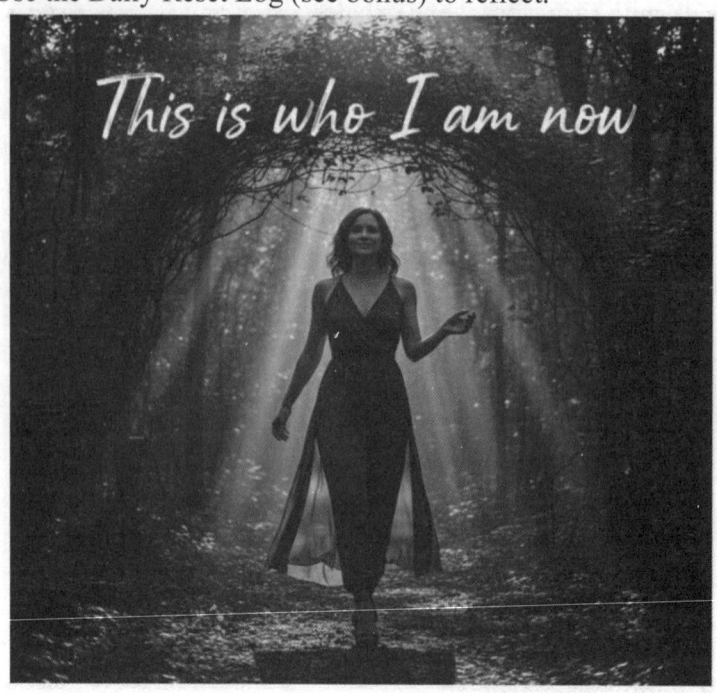

You don't need more motivation. You need a rhythm that makes you feel alive again. And it's already in your feet.

CHAPTER 8: WALKING BEYOND WEIGHT LOSS

The Spiritual and Hormonal Intelligence of Walking

When Movement Becomes Meaning.
This is not just about walking,
It's about remembering who you were before you felt broken.
It's about reawakening the woman inside who feels strong, soft, and present.

Walking Regulates Your Hormones———Silently, Powerfully.
Every step you take stimulates a cascade of hormonal balancing.
You're not just burning fat—— you're rewiring your biochemistry.

Walking:
- Lowers cortisol (stress hormone).
- Balances insulin sensitivity (key for fat metabolism).
- Boosts dopamine (motivation & joy).
- Increases oxytocin (connection & self-trust).
- Supports serotonin (emotional resilience).
- Enhances growth hormone (repair & regeneration).

Especially for women over 35, this is vital for:
Hormonal balance during peri/menopause.
PCOS regulation.
Thyroid fatigue.
Adrenal burnout.
Emotional stability.

Walking as a Moving Meditation.
The Japanese call it: Shinshin-Toitsu-"mind and body unified in action."
When you walk with awareness, the chatter of your mind begins to dissolve.
Your body becomes your spiritual anchor.
The rhythm of your steps becomes a mantra.
The breath becomes prayer.
The direction becomes purpose.
This is movement as sacred practice.

The Mirror Neuron Effect of Nature Walking.
Walking in nature activates mirror neurons tied to:
- Emotional regulation.
- Internal clarity.
- Mood elevation.
- Empathy and connection.

You become more you, because you're mirrored by the stillness and flow of the natural world.
> Trees breathe slowly.
> Water flows without force.
> Clouds move without hurry.

You begin to walk that way too.

Spiritual Walking Practices

1. The "Presence Path"
   - Walk with slow steps
   - Breath: 3:3 or 4:4
   - Every 10 steps, say silently:
   "I am here now."
   - Repeat until mind quiets

2. The Moonlight Release
   - Walk under moonlight or soft evening light
   - Visualize each exhale as release
   - Affirm:
   "With each breath, I soften."
   - Ideal for emotional shedding

3. The Gratitude Spiral
   - Start walking in circles or spiral (e. g. around a tree)
   - With each step, name one thing you're grateful for
   - Let the spiral get wider, then walk out of it Powerful when feeling disconnected or low.

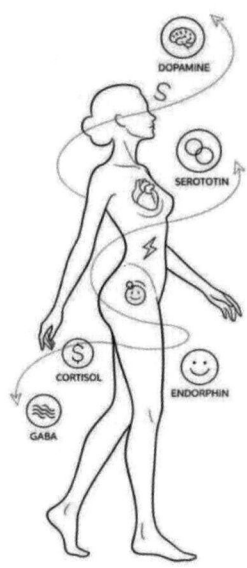

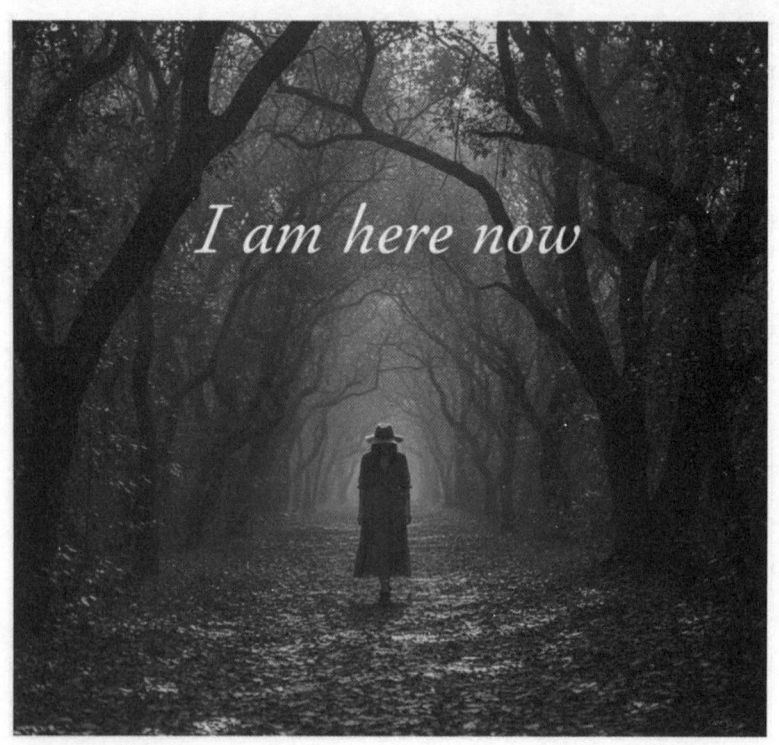

You didn't need fixing.
You needed space to move, space to breathe, and space to feel.
Walking gave you that.
And it always will.

CHAPTER 9-WALKING AS A LIFELONG HABIT

Building Your Unshakeable Walking Identity

Not just something you do. Who you become.
"I no longer need motivation.
I walk because it's who I am."

Habit vs. Identity-The Real Shift.
Most people fail to keep habits because they focus on what to do.
But transformation happens when you shift your focus to who you are becoming.
Instead of:
×"I want to walk more."
Use:
×"I am someone who walks daily, no matter what."
This small language shift rewires your brain to act in alignment with identity, not emotion.

The Habit Loop of Walking.
To make walking stick, anchor it into your neuro-habit loop:

Stage	Action
Cue	Wake up/ coffee / finish work
Routine	Walk(5-25 min)
Reward	Track steps, note energy, quick reflection

Bonus tip: Attach walking to a strong existing anchor (e. g., brushing teeth, podcast time, end of lunch).

The 5-Minute Minimum Method.
Motivation fades. Systems stick.
Set a non-negotiable minimum: just 5 minutes.

Why it works:
- Removes resistance
- Create s dopamine release upon completion
- Builds consistency muscle
- Allow s expansion (often you' ll go beyond 5)

This rewires the habit loop:→Action= Reward= Desire to repeat

Walking Identity Affirmations.
Use these after your walks or when you feel low motivation:
"I walk because I respect myself."

"Even one step makes me stronger."
"I am a woman who moves forward—— always."
"I walk to stay close to myself."
"My feet are my freedom."

Repeat them aloud, write them, or place them on your mirror.

Weekly Walking Template:
"Busy Life" Template (Time- poor days).
- Mon- Fri: 10 min breathwalk
- Sat: 25 min Flow Walk
- Sun: Optional Calm Walk

"Full Power" Template (Motivated weeks).
- Mon: Tai Chi Walking(10 min)
- Tue: JIW (3 cycles)
- Wed: breathwalk(4-6)
- Thu: Nature Flow Walk
- Fri: JIW (4-5 cycles)
- Sat: Fusion Reset
- Sun: Walk+ Journal

Optional Tools to Anchor the Habit:
- Set a daily 1- word walking reminder on phone(e. g., "BREATHE",)
- Keep a visible walking log (bonus printable provided),
- Use a ritual playlist to trigger your state,
- Assign a symbolic item (a scarf, a bracelet) as your"Walking Talisman".

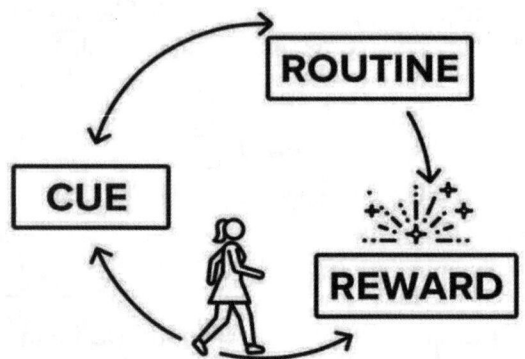

You don't need more discipline.
You need an identity you love living inside.
And step by step, that's what this book—— and your feet—— have just created.

CHAPTER 10-BONUS PROTOCOLS.

The Hidden Power Of Walking As Energy Medicine.

Bonus Techniques for Mastery, Stillness & Self- healing.
These are not exercises.
They are rituals of transformation.

QIGONG WALKING-The Ancient Flow in Motion.
What It Is:
Qigong Walking combines breath, awareness, and energetic alignment in motion. It's like meditating while you walk, and "charging" in your internal energy centers.
Benefits:
- Balances internal organs.
- Increase s"Qi"(life force).
- Releases emotional blocks.
- Improves spine alignment.
- Enhances longevity and resilience.

Basic Qigong Walking Technique-5Steps:
1. StartinWu jiposture:feethip- widt h,knees soft, arms relaxed, Inhale as you lift your right foot slowly,
2. Exhaleasyouplaceitge nt lydown ,rolling heel- to- toe.
3. Shiftweightwithawareness,feel Earth support,
4. Repeats lowly,keepingbr eathand motion synchronized.

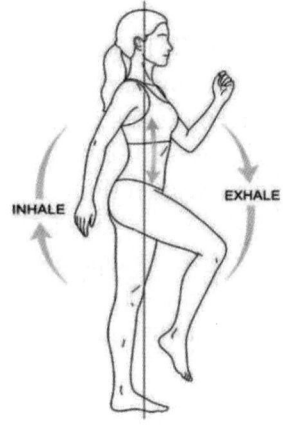

Walk in a park, barefoot if possible, ideally early morning.

Qigong Walking Vs Tai Chi Walking.

How To Blend All Three Practices For Harmony.

WHAT'S THE DIFFERENCE?
Though both Qigong Walking and Tai Chi Walking appear similar to the u ntrained eye, their intentions, energy principles, and structure are distinct. Understanding the difference helps you integrate them more intelligently.

COMPARISON TABLE:

Feature	Tai Chi Walking	Qigong Walking
Purpose	Balance, grounding, energy flow	Circulation, detox, vitality reset
Movement Speed	Very slow, fluid	Medium pace with light swinging arms
Focus Point	Structure, alignment, mindfulness	Breath coordination, relaxation
Breath Style	Deep, synced with step flow	Natural, more rhythmic and open
Arm Movement	Spiral, controlled, intentional	Loose, flowing, symmetrical
Internal Work	Strong grounding and centering(Yin)	Energetic expansion and circulation
Best Time of Day	Early morning or evening (Yin-focused)	Midday or morning (Yang-focused)
Vibe	Calm, meditative, soft power	Uplifting, restorative, flowy

HOW TO BLEND TAI CHI, QIGONG, AND JIW.
Blending the three systems gives you a 360° walking transformation: mental, emotional, physical.

Suggested Flow Structure:

Segment	Practice	Duration
1	Tai Chi Walking	10-15 min
2	Japanese Interval	15-20 min
3	Qigong Walking	10-15 min

Optional: End with Standing Meditation or Seated Breathing (3-5 min)

WHEN TO USE THIS BLEND:

You feel drained→Rebalance nervous system.
You're under high stress→Ground and circulate energy.
You need clarity→Cleanse and reset mental fog.
You want whole-body harmony→Align breath, body, and movement.

PRO TIP: Use this structure as a Weekend Reset Ritual, or a Monthly Self-Healing Practice. It's your "walking retreat"—— anytime, anywhere.

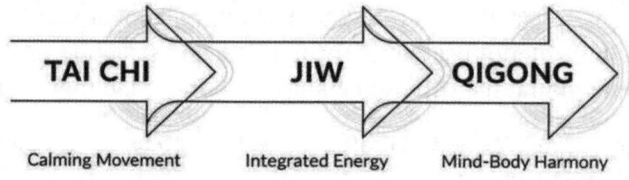

Silent Walking– The Mirror Of The Mind.

Walking in complete silence rewires the brain's default mode network, allowing for:
- Emotional integration.
- Release of overthinking.
- Heightened sensory awareness.
- Calm presence and stillness.

How to Practice:
- Walk slowly,
- No music, no phone,
- Focus on sounds of steps and environment,
- If thoughts arise, return to sensation of breath or foot contact.

Ideal for mornings, decision fatigue, or emotional overwhelm.

EMOTIONAL LOOP RESET-The Interrupt + Replace Model.
For readers trapped in repetitive emotional cycles (stress→guilt→self-doubt→paralysis),this tool creates walking-based pattern breaks.

3-Step Emotional Loop Reset:
1. Identify the Loop
    - e. g., "Every time I overeat, I feel guilty and then give up walking."
2. Interrupt It with Walking Protocol
    - Use Tai Chi Walking + 4:6 breath immediately after trigger
3. Replace It with New Emotional Anchor
    Affirm:"I walk to release, not to punish."

Walk becomes therapy→breaks conditioned response →rewires neuro-association.

Summary Chart: Bonus Protocols:

Technique	Goal	Best Time
Qigong Walking	Energize, balance	Morning or after illness
Silent Walk	Emotional integration	Mornings / post-stress
Emotional Loop Reset	Behavior shift	After triggers or setbacks

You have learned how to walk.
Now you know how to breathe.
Now you know how to feel while walking.
What's next?
Keep walking—— as who you' ve become.

30-DAY HEALING WALK PLAN (CALENDAR)

This is a progressive 4-week walking transformation plan structured as:

Week	Theme	Focus
1	Awareness	Breathing, posture, body scan
2	Rhythm	Cadence, pace variation, musical sync
3	Energy	Chi flow, mental clarity, vitality
4	Integration	All-in-one: Tai Chi + JIW + Qigong

Each day includes a purpose-driven walk, with short prompts or focus exercises.

WEEK1:AWARENESS(Days 1-7)

Goal: Reconnect mind and body through slow, conscious walking.

Day	Focus	Instructions
1	Breathing Awareness	Walk 15 mins focusing only on nose breathing.
2	Posture Alignment	Use wall posture drill before walk; hold spine upright.
3	Slow Walking Meditation	Walk at half your normal pace, noticing foot contact.
4	Grounding Steps	Visualize roots with each step. Barefoot if possible.
5	Body Scan Walking	Move attention through your body as you walk.
6	Visual Focus Technique	Gaze at the horizon during walk. No devices.
7	Stillness Start	Begin walk with 2m ins standing still, eyes closed.

WEEK2:RHYTHM(Days 8-14)

Goal: Establish your unique walking rhythm with breath, music, and pace.

Day	Focus	Instructions
8	Natural Rhythm Check	Walk without music. Observe your natural cadence.
9	Cadence Counting	Count steps for 30 seconds, repeat.
10	Music Match BPM	Walk to a song at 90–100 BPM. Sync steps.
11	Interval Start(20/10)	Walk 20 secs fast / 10 secs slow x10 rounds.
12	Arm Swing Coordination	Sync your arms to your step rhythm.
13	3-Step Breathing	Inhale 3 steps, exhale 3 steps.
14	Beat Walking	Use music to dictate pace(playlist suggested in Bonus).

WEEK3:E NERGY(Days 15-21)

Goal: Increase chi circulation, inner vitality, and oxygen efficiency.

Day	Focus	Instructions
15	Chi Ball Visualization	Imagine holding a ball of energy while walking.
16	Energy Fingers	Walk with fingertips gently open, sensing air.
17	Reverse Breathing	Inhale as belly contracts, exhale it expands.
18	Shoulder Loosening	Add gentle shoulder rotations during walk.
19	Qigong Arm Swings	Walk with rhythmic swinging arms (see Bonus 1).
20	Mental Affirmations	Repeat "I move with energy and calm."
21	Gratitude Walk	Focus on what you're thankful for with each step.

WEEK4: INTEGRATION (Days 22-30)

Goal: Blend Tai Chi Walking, Japanese Interval Walking, and Qigong into one intuitive practice.

Day	Focus	Instructions
22	Tai Chi Walk Sequence	10 min practice of Core Form (see Chapter 7)
23	JIW 15/15 Style	Alternate 15 sec fast/ 15 sec slow x20
24	Nature+ Stillness Combo	Walk in green space, pause 5 times to breathe deeply.
25	Healing Walk Flow	Combine posture, breath, rhythm, silence.
26	Qigong Opening-Walk-Closing	Begin with Qigong stance, walk, end with closing palms.
27	Community Sync (if possible)	Walk with a friend or family, in silence.
28	Sunrise Energy Walk	Wake early, walk facing rising sun.
29	All-in-One Loop	5min Tai Chi +10 min JIW+ 5m in Qigong.
30	Celebration Walk	Reflect on your month. Walk with your favorite music.

CHAPTER 11: How To Teach Others & Form Walking Groups.

Why Teach or Walk in Groups?
One of the most powerful ways to deepen your healing walk practice is to share it. Teaching others not only reinforces your own understanding, but also builds community, accountability, and emotional support—— all essential ingredients for long-term wellness. Whether you want to guide a small circle of friends or organize a local walking group, this section gives you the exact structure to do it with confidence.

Benefits of Group Walking Practice:
    Motivation & Accountability——People show up for each other.
    Shared Learning—— Everyone brings insight and energy.
    Emotional Support—— Deep conversations happen on walks.
    Consistency—— Routine walks help habits stick.
    Leadership Growth—— You become a positive influence in others' lives.

How to Start Teaching or Leading.

1. Know Your Practice First.
Only lead what you truly understand. Start by mastering the Tai Chi Walking basics and Japanese Interval structure from this book.

2. Choose Your Format:

Format	Description
1-on-1	Ideal for friends, family, or clients
Small Group	3–6 people, perfect for quiet parks or trails
Workshop	60-90 minute session with theory + practice
Weekly Meetup	Ongoing group with a set time, e. g. every Saturday at 9 AM

3. Pick a Location:
    Flat walking trail, park loop, or community track,
    Low noise, nature preferred,
    Accessible for all ages.

4. Create a Simple Structure.
Here's a sample format for a 45-minute group walk:

Time	Activity
0-5m in	Centering (posture + breath)
5–10 min	Tai Chi Walking warm-up
10–25 min	Japanese Interval rounds (e. g., 10/10 or 15/15)
25-40 min	Gentle Qigong walking
40–45 min	Cooldown & reflection (standing or seated)

How to Lead a Simple Introduction.
" Welcome Today we' ll explore a fusion of gentle movement and mindful breath that improves energy, balance, and emotional calm. You don't need experience —— just your breath, body, and an open mind."
Then guide them step-by-step using the instructions inside this book.

Tips for Success:
- Start with friends or family before advertising publicly,
- Always demonstrate before asking others to move,
- Speak calmly, clearly, with pauses,
- Keep the mood open, not perfectionist,
- Allow questions, but avoid long lectures,
- Use a Bluetooth speaker (low volume) for music if desired,
- Encourage journaling or shared reflection post-walk.

Sample Group Invite Text (Customizable).
"Join our Weekly healing Walk Group"
Every Saturday | 9 AM | Park entrance near Maple Grove
Experience the benefits of Tai Chi Walking, Japanese Intervals, and breath Movement.
Beginners welcome. Free and peaceful.
RSVP to [your email or group link]

BONUS-WALKING JOURNAL TEMPLATE
Track, Reflect, Review

Why a Walking Journal Changes Everything.
"You don't know what you've changed,
until you write it down."
Tracking your walks isn't about discipline —— it's about witnessing your own transformation in real time.

A journal:
    Shows how far you've come,
    Gives you motivation on hard days,
    Keeps the habit alive,
    Creates a loop of success + emotional memory,
    Turns abstract benefits into visible proof.

How to Use Your Walking Journal.
Each page =1 day. Fill it in after your walk (or during your cool-down).
No pressure. No perfection. Just presence.

Daily Walk Journal Template:

Section	Prompt
Date	(Fill in)
Walk Type	Tai Chi/JIW/ Breathwalk/ Flow/ etc.
Duration	(Minutes walked)
My Focus Word	e. g., "Clarity", "Peace", "Power"
What I Noticed	A feeling, a sound, a thought
My Emotion Now	Calm/ Energized/ Hopeful/ etc.
Insight or Gratitude	e. g., "I felt my body again."

Journal Page Template

My Walking Journey

DATE

TIME / DURATION

DISTANCE / ROUTE

THOUGHTS / MOOD

DAILY REFLECTION
THE EARTH HAS MUSIC FOR THOSE WHO LISTEN.

How To Use Bpm To Boost The Power Of Your Healing Walks.

WHY BPM MATTERS (BPM = Beats Per Minute).
Just like heart rate, music tempo affects your pace, energy output, and rhythm. Scientific studies on Japanese Interval Walking show that matching music tempo to walking effort improves:
- Fat burn,
- Endurance,
- Focus and motivation,
- Walking posture and rhythm.

INTERVAL MUSIC SYNCING.

Use this BPM-based structure during your Japanese Interval Walks (JIW):

PHASE	BPM RANGE	MUSIC STYLE
Warm-up	90-100	Ambient, soft piano
Fast Walking	120-140	Funk, Pop, Uplifting EDM
Slow Recovery	80-100	Chillhop, Lo-fi, Soft Jazz

EXAMPLE INTERVAL: "10-MIN WALK CYCLE".
1. 2min-Warm-up (Lo-fi at 95 BPM),
2. 2min-Fast Interval (Pop at 130 BPM),
3. 1min-Recovery (Soft Jazz at 85 BPM),
4. Repeat x2.

PRO TIP: Let the music "pull" your stride.
When the beat matches your ideal walking cadence (ex:130 steps per min), you'll enter a natural rhythm = longer duration, less fatigue.

SUGGESTED SPOTIFY PLAYLISTS
(Search for these on Spotify by name)
- Healing Walk Focus-90 BPM
- Interval Burn-130 BPM High Energy
- Tai Chi Zen Flow-Meditative 60-70 BPM
- Qigong Breath Rhythm-Grounding Lo-fi
- Sunrise Reset-Mixed BPM for Harmony

Or Create Your Own: Use walk.bpmtools.com or getsongbpm.com
These free tools help find music by BPM for each phase of your walk.

HOW TO TEACH OTHERS & FORM WALKING GROUPS
Spread The Practice, Build The Community, Elevate The healing

Once you've experienced the benefits of Tai Chi Walking, Japanese Interval Walking, andQigong Walking, the natural step is to share it. Whether with friends, your neighborhood, or a small class, you can lead others gently and confidently, even if you're not a certified teacher.

WHY TEACH OTHERS?
> Reinforces your own practice,
> Create s motivation and accountability,
> Deepens emotional connection and purpose,
> Allow s you to be a force for wellness in your circle,
> Elevates your confidence and voice.

Teaching is the biggest form of learning. When you guide, you integrate.

START SMALL: THE "MICRO-CLASS" METHOD.
You don't need a studio or license to begin. Try this simple structure:

Phase	Time	What to Do
1. Welcome	3-5min	Ask about energy levels, mood, intentions
2. Warm-Up	5m in	Simple Qigong arm swings, breathing in place
3. Practice	15-20 min	Choose 1: Tai Chi walk, JIW cycle, or 10/10/10
4. Cool Down	5min	Qigong walk or standing breathing
5. Sharing	3min	Ask: "What did you feel?" or "One word to describe today"

FORMING A WALKING GROUP:
Where to begin:
> Start with 1-2 friends,
> Use a WhatsApp app or Facebook event,
> Choose a recurring time (ex: Sunday 9am),
> Meet at a local park or open space,
> Keep it simple: walking shoes, water bottle, open heart

Best group types:
> Stress Recovery Circles (Tai Chi + Qigong focus),
> Active Wellness Clubs (JIW + BPM playlists),
> Mixed Energy Walks (rotate all three styles weekly).

LEADER TIPS (No certification needed).
> Speak clearly, gently, and from your own experience,
> Demonstrate slowly —— use your body, not technical words,
> Focus on energy, presence, rhythm —— not perfection,
> Let silence be part of the session,
> Always ask for consent if offering physical guidance.

PRO TIP: Use this script to invite people.

" Hi I'm starting a gentle walking group to improve balance, energy, and mood. It's beginner- friendly, calming,and powerful. Want to join us for a free 30- min walk this weekend?"

REFERENCES: Studies, Sources, and Traditions.

This book is inspired by and built upon decades of traditional Eastern walking practices,modern exercise physiology, and behavioral neuroscience. The following sources, research,and historical insights were referenced and adapted into the healing Walk Fusion method:

Tai Chi Walking
- Gallwey, J.& Hegner, C. Tai Chi Walking: A Low-Impact Path to BetterHealth, Strength, and Balance
- Wolfe, D. Tai Chi Walking for Beginners: Mindfulness in Motion
- National Center for Complementary and Integrative Health (NCCIH):Tai Chi and Qi Walking for Health
- Harvard Health Publishing: The health benefits of Tai Chi
- Traditional Yang-Style and Wu-Style Tai Chi movement frameworks.

Japanese Interval Walking (JIW)
- Matsuo, T., et al. Effects of High-Intensity Interval Walking on Fat Loss and Cardiovascular Health, Japanese Society of Physical Fitness
- NHK Japan and Japanese Ministry of Health promotional content on"Interval Walking"
- NHK World-Japan, Science View documentary (2023)

Qigong Walking
- Institute of Integral Qigong and Tai Chi (IIQTC)
- Janka, H. Walking Qigong: Harmonizing Body and breath
- Lao Tzu's Tao Te Ching-Philosophical foundations for breath-based movement
- Chen-style and Medical Qigong variants for mobility

Mind-Body & Behavior Science
- Dr. Andrew Huberman, Huberman Lab-The Neuroscience of Habit &Movement
- Dr. Kelly McGonigal-The Joy of Movement
- WHO Guidelines on Physical Activity (2022 revision)
- Harvard School of Public Health-Benefits of Moderate IntensityWalking
- NIH: Cognitive and Emotional Benefits of Walking Daily

These references were adapted and translated into practical, accessible guidance for readers of all levels and backgrounds. We acknowledge that some of the traditional knowledge passed down is oral and ancestral, not always traceable to single authors or publications.

Cultural Acknowledgments.

We honor and respectfully acknowledge the deep cultural and historical roots of the practices included in this book:

> Tai Chi and Qigong originate from ancient Chinese martial and healing arts, cultivated through generations in Taoist, Buddhist, and Confucian traditions. We thank the global Tai Chi and Qigong communities for preserving and evolving these arts with integrity and compassion.
> Japanese Interval Walking draws from a unique blend of scientific innovation and cultural reverence for daily motion as a pillar of health inJapan. We are inspired by the Japanese ethos of kaizen (continuous improvement), ikigai (life purpose), and the disciplined lifestyle of active aging.

We do not claim to replace or replicate traditional instruction, but rather aim to honor these traditions by offering a respectful, modern fusion that empowersWestern readers through structured, accessible, and safe practice.

To the masters, researchers, and practitioners before us: thank you for lighting the path.

♥ Final Words To The Reader
You didn't just buy a book.
You chose a new rhythm. A new breath. A new story.
And every single step you take...
tells the world:
"I am walking back to myself."